THE New York State Lunatic Asylum at UTICA

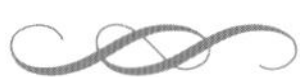

A HISTORY OF OLD MAIN

DENNIS WEBSTER

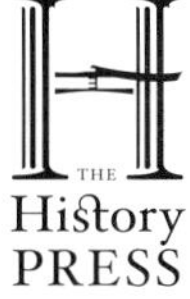

Published by The History Press
Charleston, SC
www.historypress.com

First published 2021

Manufactured in the United States

ISBN 9781467148429

Library of Congress Control Number: 2021937212

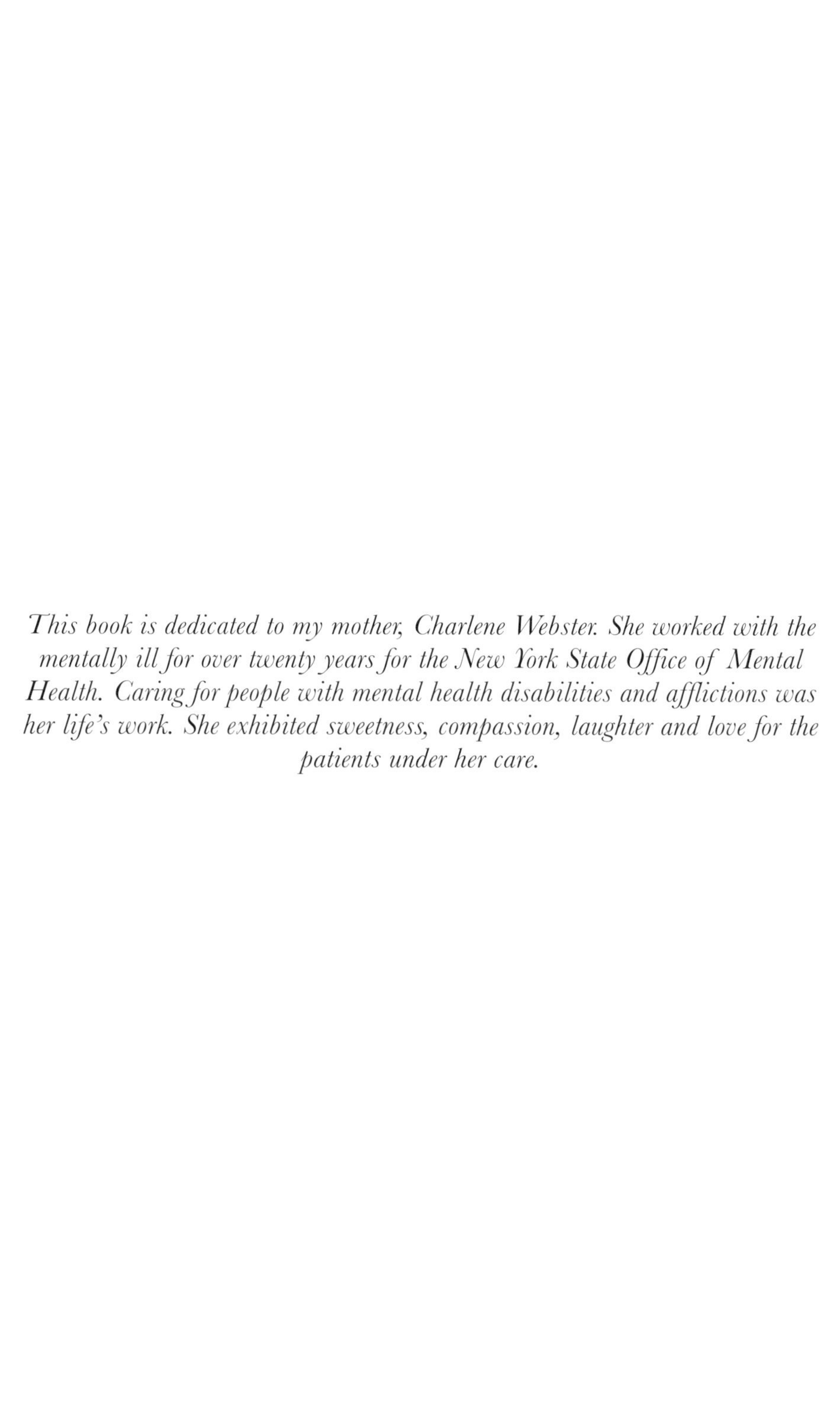

This book is dedicated to my mother, Charlene Webster. She worked with the mentally ill for over twenty years for the New York State Office of Mental Health. Caring for people with mental health disabilities and afflictions was her life's work. She exhibited sweetness, compassion, laughter and love for the patients under her care.

Contents

Foreword

The New York State Lunatic Asylum at Utica. The Utica Psychiatric Center. The Mohawk Valley Psychiatric Center Building No. 31. Old Main.

No matter what it's been called over time, no other building in the Greater Utica area holds such intrigue, mystery, both architectural and historical awe, fondness and yes, even loathing as does the structure we now know as Old Main. For many years, this facility was a solid employer, with a building and associated campus that defined the Highland area of West Utica since it opened in 1841. Many people have memories of working there or had friends or relatives who did or darker memories of loved ones who were patients there. It embodies the history of the innovative treatment of the mentally ill from when it first opened until it closed. To recognize its place in local, state and national history, Old Main is not only listed in the National Register of Historic Places but also designated as a National Historic Landmark (NHL) for its architectural and historical significance and also for the individuals who were associated with its design and operation. Listing as an NHL is the highest designation that can be afforded a building. There are only two in Utica; the other is the Miller-Conkling-Kernan House at 3 Rutger Park.

When Old Main closed, this huge building no longer had a function. This is where the Landmarks Society of Greater Utica comes in. Formed in 1974, Landmarks long recognized the critical importance of this monumental structure and the real threat that it faced when it closed due

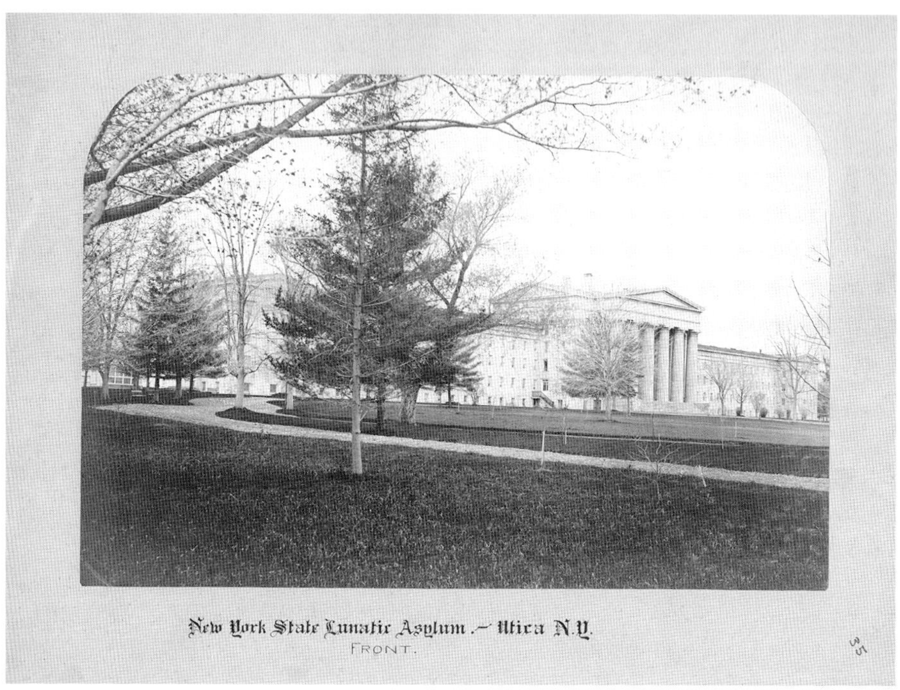

Front view of the Lunatic Asylum. *New York State Archives.*

to the changed treatment model that rejected large institutional buildings like this one. The society remained vigilant in keeping Old Main in the public eye and strongly advocated for much-needed improvements to keep it weathertight while a new use was sought for it. Several years after Old Main closed, the state invested over $2 million, as a direct result of the efforts of the Landmarks Society, for a new roof, new gutters and rebuilding the imposing limestone front steps, even though the building was unoccupied and with no new use identified.

While Old Main remained essentially mothballed, in 1999 a new threat surfaced. The Preservation League of New York State informed us that the state proposed to sell "surplus buildings," and that Old Main was on that list. The Landmarks Society formed the Old Main Redevelopment Advisory Committee to directly address this potential threat, as a buyer might not understand or appreciate its historical and architectural significance. We also actively sought a compatible adaptive reuse.

Those efforts paid off. The state took Old Main off of its for sale list, sought out and obtained a Save America's Treasures matching grant, undertook a significant restoration of the ground-floor entry and office area and converted the remainder of the first floor into a New York State Office of Mental Health (OMH) records storage facility. Restoration and reuse efforts continue under OMH's stewardship.

The Landmarks Society remains the most significant and stalwart advocate for Old Main. In August 2014, with the permission and cooperation of the NYS OMH and as part of its Summer Walks and Talks series, a tour of the first floor of Old Main was offered that drew literally thousands of people.

It is the fervent hope of the Landmarks Society that the state will continue to use and care for this monumentally important facility and that someday a museum could be located in the central portion of Old Main that is dedicated to the vast (and sometimes painful) history of the treatment of the mentally ill and once again regain worldwide significance and recognition. In the meantime, please enjoy this insightful historical view of this fascinating structure.

—Michael J. Bosak
Vice President (Education)
The Landmarks Society of Greater Utica
November 2020

Preface

I want the reader to know that I put the greatest care into the research into this book and in no way judge the people, who, at the time, tried their best to provide proper care to the mentally ill. Like any medical treatment, advances in technology and increased intellectual capital into maladies have improved in each successive generation. Utica, and the surrounding communities of the Mohawk Valley, are proud and fond of Old Main, and this book is meant to be for them and others who might not know the details of the asylum. The Old Main structure has been viewed fondly by the people in Utica since its birth, and the fascination continues today with throngs of people coming out for tours. The fight to stem the decay and the disappearance of Old Main is underway. May the grand structure stand in infinity and continue to remind and inspire those of the current generation.

Introduction

The Lunatic Asylum at Utica, fondly referred to as "Old Main," is among a smattering of buildings on a sprawling campus on the western edge of the city of Utica, New York. The Old Main building is the centerpiece and the structure most identified with psychiatric care in New York State. Old Main opened its doors to patients on January 16, 1843. At that time, it was one of the first lunatic asylums in the United States. New York State had one small facility, the Bloomingdale Asylum, which housed a small, segmented population of the insane. Old Main would be the first asylum in the United States that would house people with all types of mental illnesses, from the entire state of New York, and would offer moral treatment that was prevalent in Europe but unknown on our shores. Previously, people with mental illness were locked away in basements, attics or prisons, where they would be shackled in irons. Hidden away from public view and forgotten with no hope.

In the annals of Oneida County, there is an account of the care of patients before the asylum was built. The following was taken from a mid-nineteenth-century publication:

> *The insane had been treated as the forsaken of God, in whom the evil spirit had taken up his abode. They were chained in cages and dungeons, without attendance, without clothing, fire or wholesome food, suffering from cold, heat, impure air, filth and vermin; in solitude and darkness; with no sounds but the clanking of their chains, the rattling of the bars and grates and their own shrieks, curses and moans; with never a kind word or look, and never*

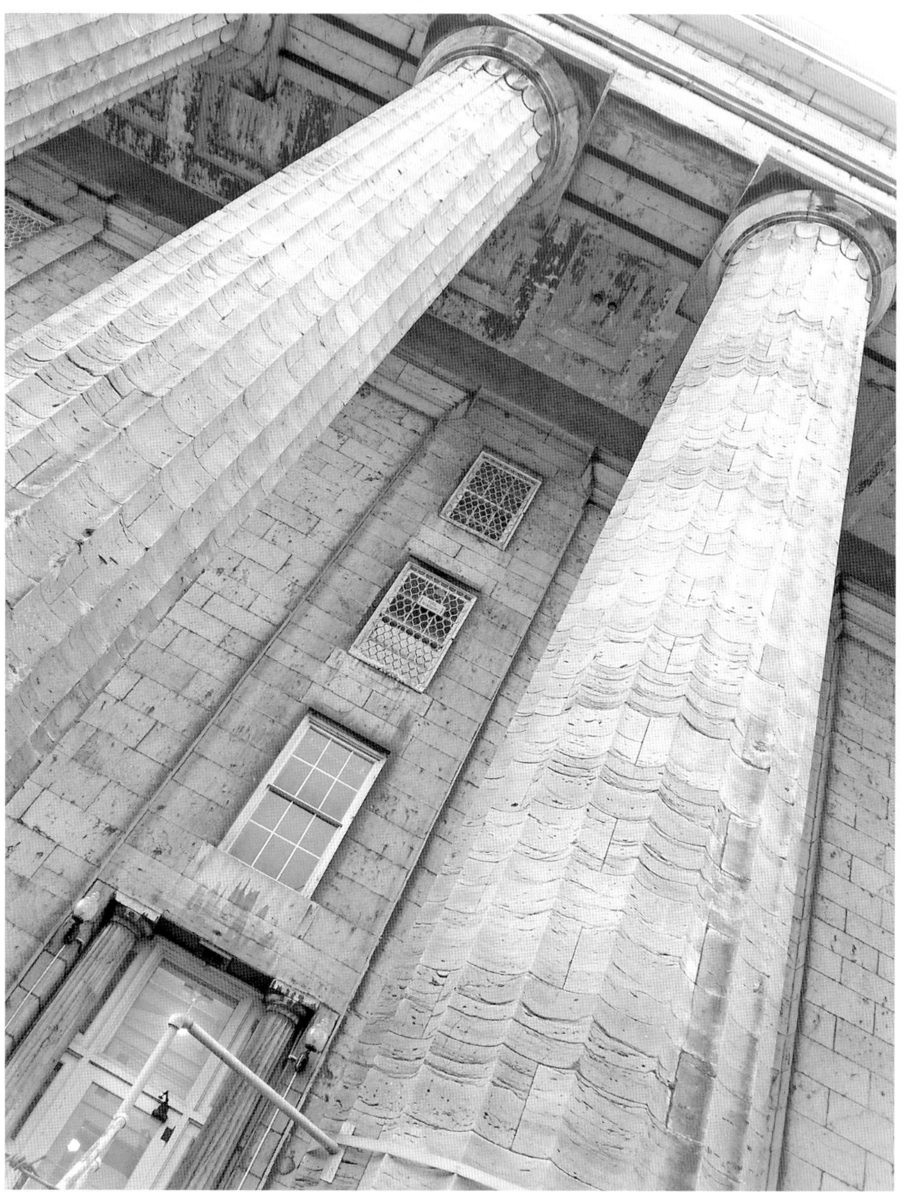

visited but to be taunted and tormented, and teased to be made to exhibit the frenzy and power of the maniac—until nature was worn out, may be after many years—and death more kind than man, came to the relief of the sufferer, and earth was relieved of a burden and disgrace and his friends of a reproach. What a change!

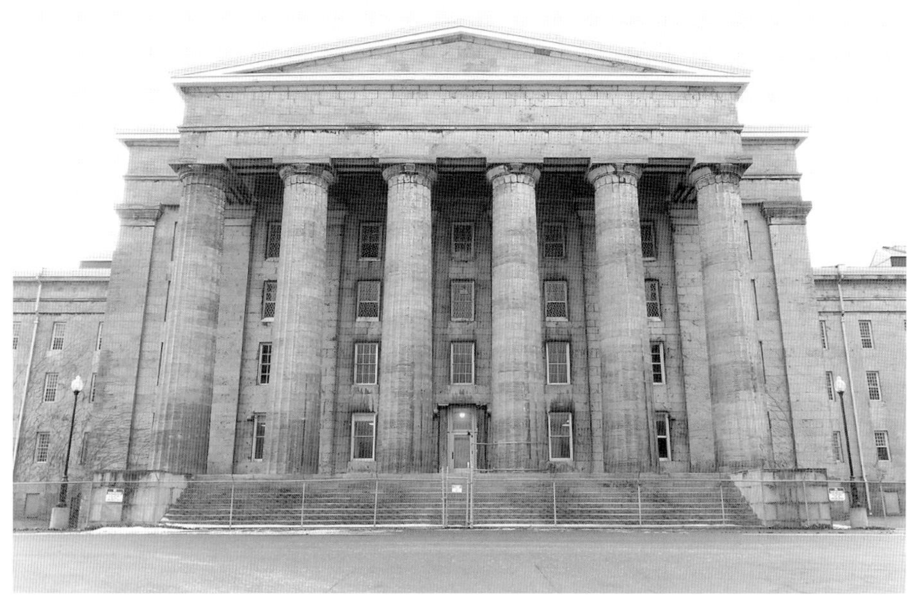

Opposite: The Greek Doric columns loom large. *New York State Archives.*

Above: The beautiful and grand Greek Doric front entrance to Old Main. *Courtesy Jeff Berman.*

The Lunatic Asylum at Utica represented a new beginning in the care and treatment of those with mental illnesses. The first administrator was Dr. Amariah Brigham, who had been inspired by Philippe Pinel (1745–1826). At the end of the eighteenth century, people who were considered lunatics or mentally insane were treated with much disdain by even the most civilized of European countries. Even in the United States of America, people with mental illness were chained in basements or locked in jails to be forever hidden from public view. They were forgotten human beings with no quality of life, no chance of release and manacled with iron chains, bound to brick and mortar until their tortured souls departed their rotten, dead and neglected bodies. Pinel would change this. Philippe Pinel was born in France and is credited with the "moral treatment" in the care of those with mental illness. Before Pinel, lunatics were chained to walls of dark dungeons and believed to be possessed by the devil. They would sometimes be flogged, beaten, displayed like circus animals for money without any hope of release. Doomed to a lifetime of hell on earth. Pinel became the superintendent of the Bicetre Insane Asylum in Paris, France, in 1792. He unchained the

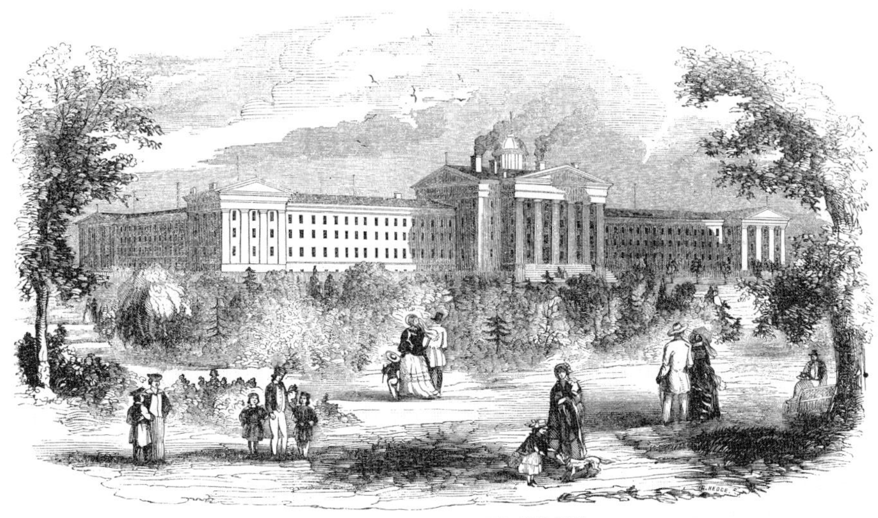

Artist rendering of the exterior picturesque Gothic landscaping. *Oneida County History Center.*

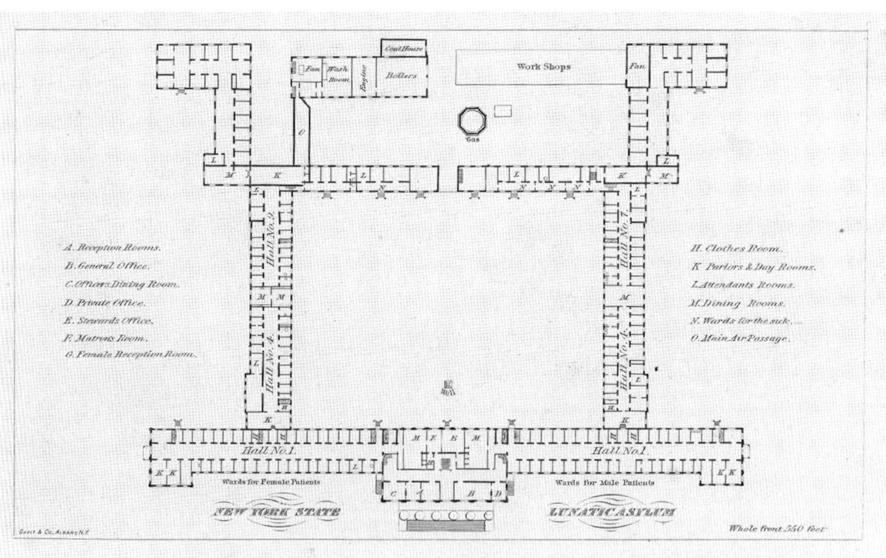

Lunatic Asylum original floor plan. The design had called for the wings to be enclosed, providing a thirteen-acre courtyard. This plan was never completed due to lack of funds. *New York State Archives.*

New York State Lunatic Asylum.- Utica N.Y.
END VIEW WITH GREEN HOUSE.
36

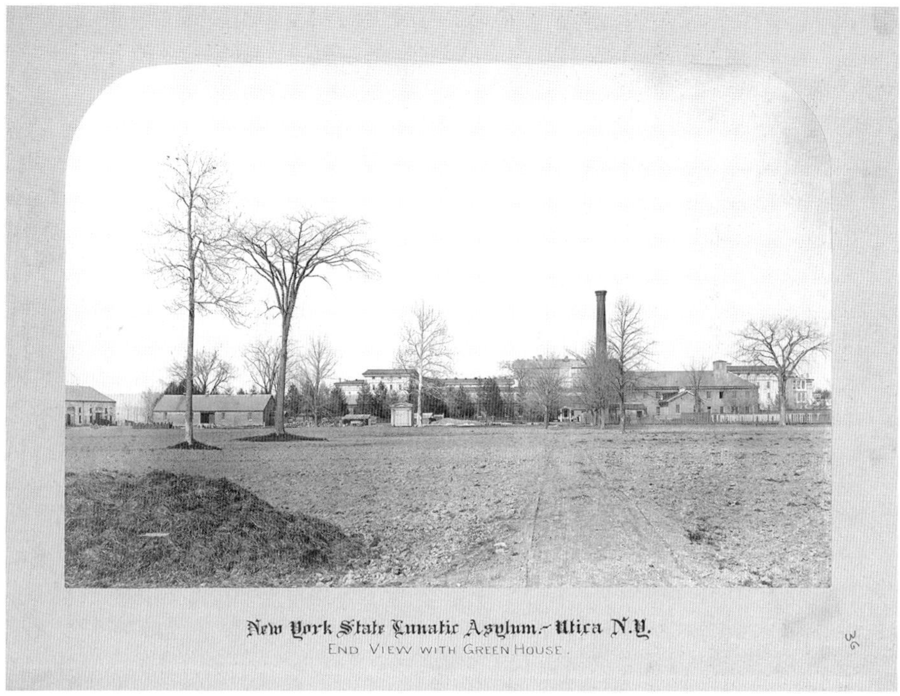

End view of the Lunatic Asylum. *New York State Archives.*

lunatics, discussed with them their mental illnesses and offered classes in self-control and normality. The social skills and rehabilitation of the insane was a remarkable achievement that made Pinel an international celebrity, and he is now called the father of modern psychiatry.

When the patients at the Lunatic Asylum at Utica, in 1850, decided to write and edit their own periodical, the *Opal*, they used an image of Pinel to grace the front cover. Dr. Amariah Brigham would pattern the care at the Lunatic Asylum at Utica, which opened in 1843, after Pinel's moral treatment in an attempt to provide a Utopian experience for the mentally ill. One innovation was the use of religion as therapy. Church attendance was mandatory for all patients except those most severe cases who were placed in Utica cribs (restraining devices with locking lids). The church services were overseen by Reverend Chauncey E. Goodrich from 1843 to 1863. According to Benjamin Reiss, in *Theaters of Madness*, when Old Main opened, the doctors of the time considered insanity "a chronic disease of the brain, producing either derangement of the intellectual faculties, or prolonged change of the feelings, affections, and habits of an individual."

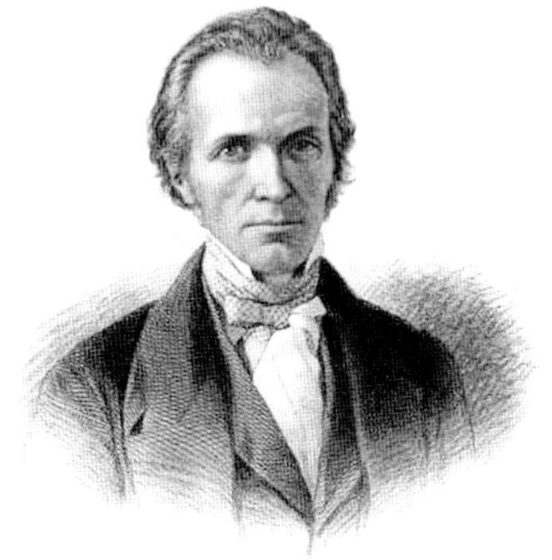

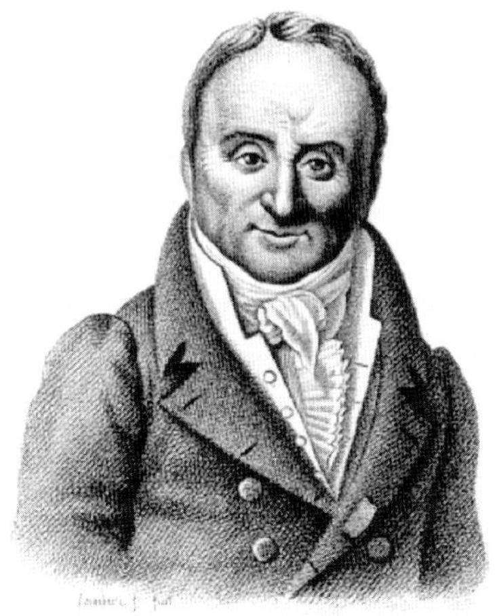

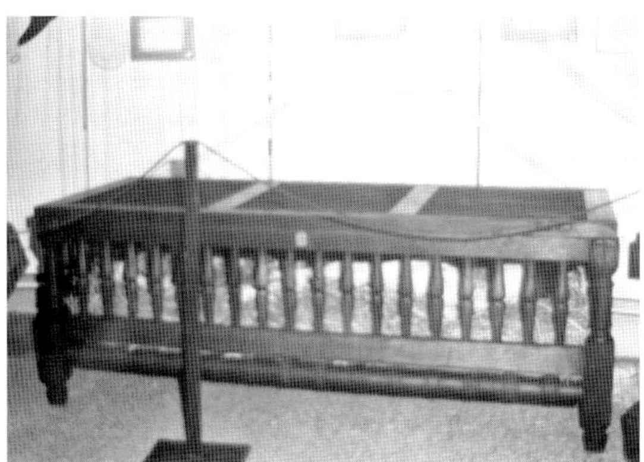

Above, left: Dr. Amariah Brigham was the first superintendent of the Lunatic Asylum at Utica, New York. *Oneida County History Center.*

Above, right: Philippe Pinel (1745–1826) started moral treatment for the insane in France in the eighteenth century. *Oneida County History Center*.

Left: Utica crib on display. *New York State Archives*.

Old Main may have some subject matter and phrasing that is sure to offend and shock. I urge the reader to close the book, set it down and walk away if such descriptions may foul your morality or violate your sensibilities. Everything must be looked at in the time it occurred: different generations, words, actions, therapies and devices. The treatment was not meant to be barbaric, especially with the application of the Utica crib. In the mid-nineteenth century, that device was invented and introduced with great admiration as a new, modern way to treat those with mental illness. Those who arrived at the asylum in chains would have them removed before they stepped foot inside the building. It's no different with things like lobotomy, electroshock therapy, restraints both physical and chemical. This book is meant to inform and not stand in judgment of those who, at the time, were trying the best methods to treat those with mental illness. The

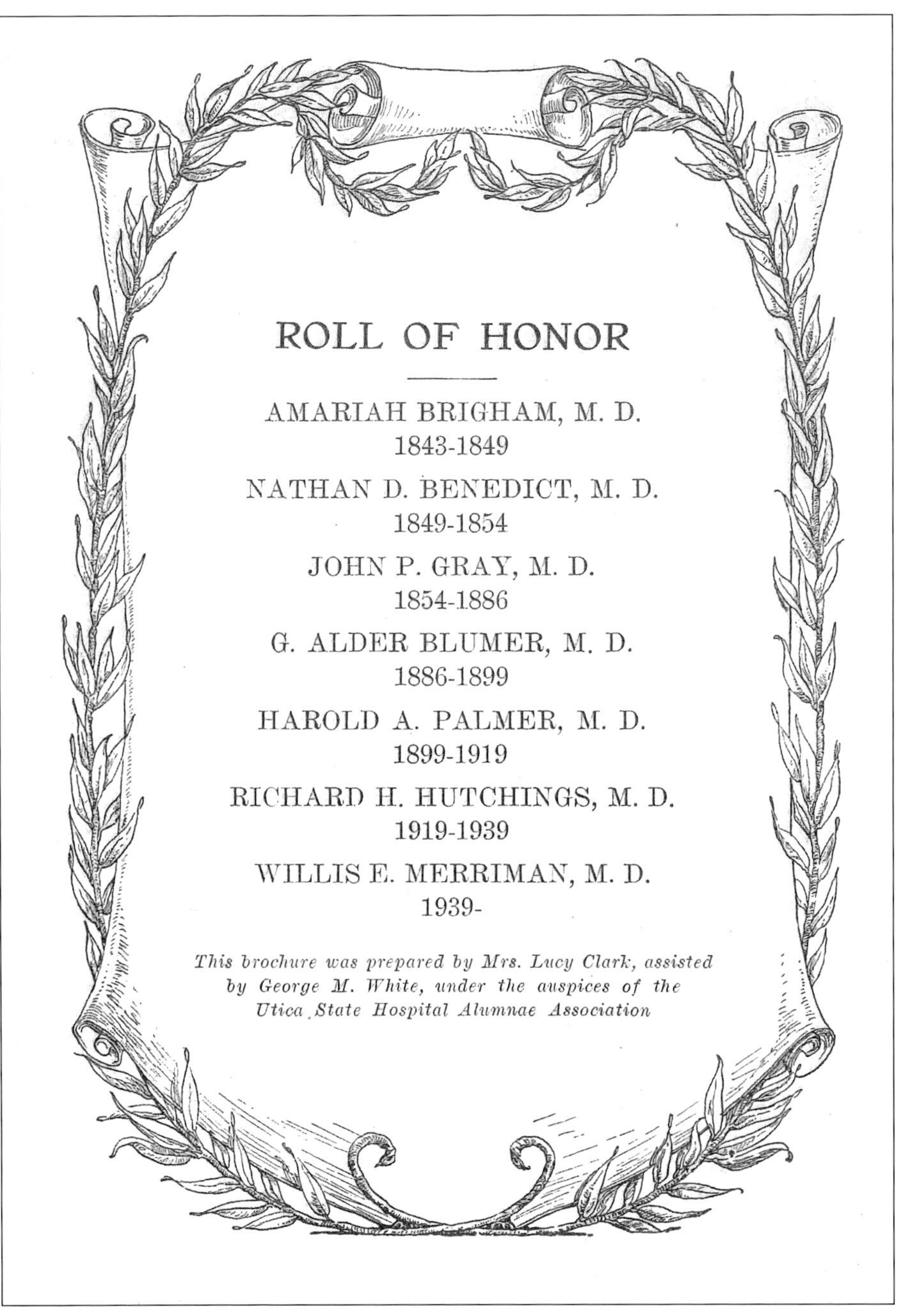
ROLL OF HONOR

AMARIAH BRIGHAM, M. D.
1843-1849

NATHAN D. BENEDICT, M. D.
1849-1854

JOHN P. GRAY, M. D.
1854-1886

G. ALDER BLUMER, M. D.
1886-1899

HAROLD A. PALMER, M. D.
1899-1919

RICHARD H. HUTCHINGS, M. D.
1919-1939

WILLIS E. MERRIMAN, M. D.
1939-

This brochure was prepared by Mrs. Lucy Clark, assisted by George M. White, under the auspices of the Utica State Hospital Alumnae Association

The first seven superintendents of Old Main. *Oneida County History Center.*

Lunatic Asylum gave way to the name Utica State Hospital and then Utica Psychiatric Center and delivered patient care from 1843 until its closure to patients in 1978 when safety code violations led to transfer to other buildings on the campus.

OLD MAIN SUPERINTENDENTS

Amariah Brigham, MD (1843–1849)
Nathan D. Benedict, MD (1849–1854)
John P. Gray, MD (1854–1886)
G. Alder Blumer, MD (1886–1899)
Harold A. Palmer, MD (1899–1919)
Richard H. Hutchings, MD (1919–1939)
Willis E. Merriman, MD (1939–1946)
Arthur W. Pense, MD (1946–1948)
Harold A. Pooler, MD (1948–1949)
Francis J. O'Neill, MD (1949–1951)
Bascomb B. Young, MD (1951–1959)
Martin Lazar, MD (1959–1963)
George Volow, MD (1963–1976)
Nelson Sanchez, MD (1976–1977)
Richard M. Heath (1977–1992)

Old Main closed in 1978. The Utica Psychiatric Center consolidated under Marcy State Hospital in 1976, and both were supervised by a single superintendent.

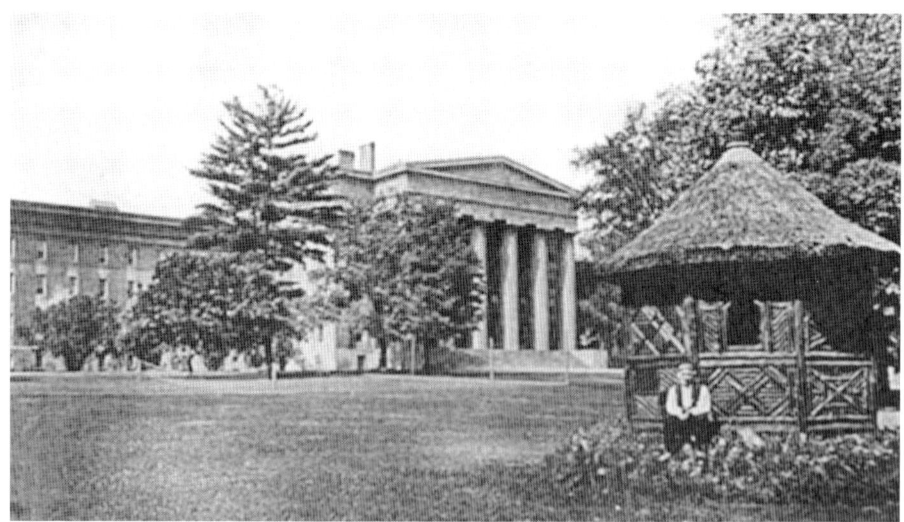

Front view of Old Main with gazebo. *Oneida County History Center.*

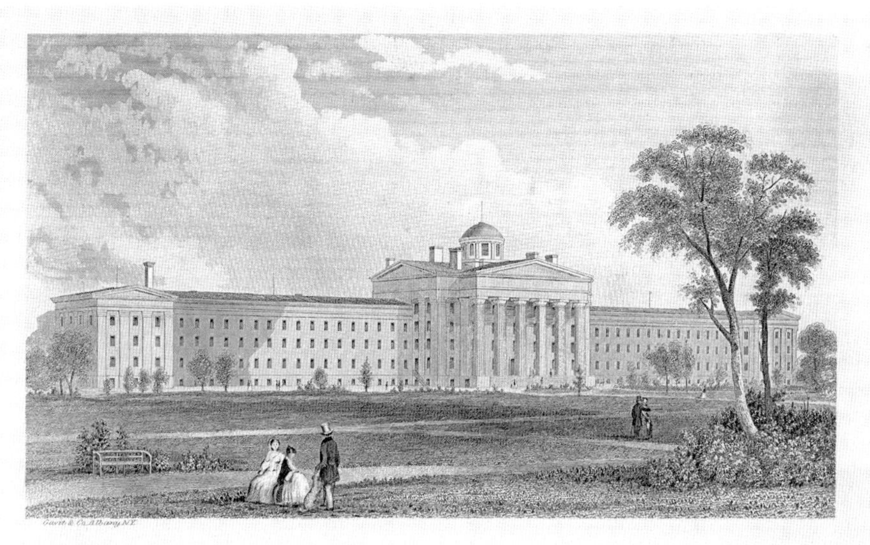

The Empire State built the asylum to showcase the Utopian care provided within. *New York State Archives.*

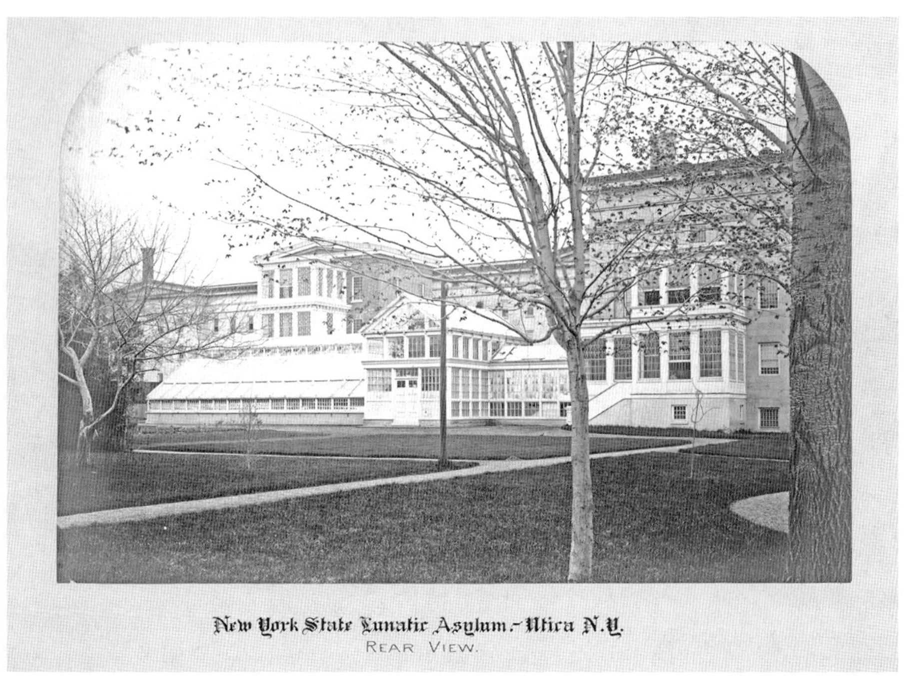

Rear view of the Lunatic Asylum. *New York State Archives.*

THE CITY OF UTICA AND THE MOHAWK VALLEY

Old Main was built on the western edge of the city of Utica, New York. The first location that New York State considered was a tract of farmland in Watervliet. A disagreement with the property owner forced the state to seek another location, and the emerging city of Utica was chosen for its beautiful location and proximity to the Erie Canal and Chenango Canal. A location on the western edge of Utica was purchased for $10,000, but the 130 acres required additional funds, so citizens raised another $6,300 to complete the purchase. Utica is situated in the midst of the Mohawk Valley of Central New York, where the most gorgeous scenery and rustic beauty exist on the entire planet. It made sense to place a Utopian asylum in the midst of the mist of this Garden of Eden.

Part I

New York State Lunatic Asylum at Utica (1843–1889)

Amariah Brigham, MD (1843–1849)

Dr. Brigham was the first superintendent of the New York State Lunatic Asylum at Utica. His innovations included bringing occupations to the patients. He viewed it as healthy to the mind to work and have purpose. He had a working farm that had chickens, horses, pigs and cows along with a vegetable garden, a beehive and a print shop. Jobs included carpentry, kitchen duties such as meal preparation, cleaning, seamstress work and many others. Instead of chaining people to walls, he put them to work. Dr. Brigham used Shaker methodologies, which included a very strict day. (The Shakers were a Christian sect known for strict rules, including mode of dress.) Bells would ring when patients were to rise from bed, go to meals, go to bed and go to church. Everyone had to wear Shaker-style clothing, and it was laundered every day along with the bedding. Dr. Brigham started the *American Journal of Insanity* in 1844 in the print shop and invented the Utica crib. Amariah Brigham was born on December 26, 1798, in New Marlborough, Massachusetts. When he was eleven years old, his father passed away, so Amariah went to live with his uncle in Schoharie, New York. Amariah dreamed of being a physician—as his uncle was one of high regard—but when Amariah was fourteen years old, his uncle passed away. The lad went to Albany to live on his own. Eventually, he went back to Massachusetts to live with his mother and started to study under physicians. He became a

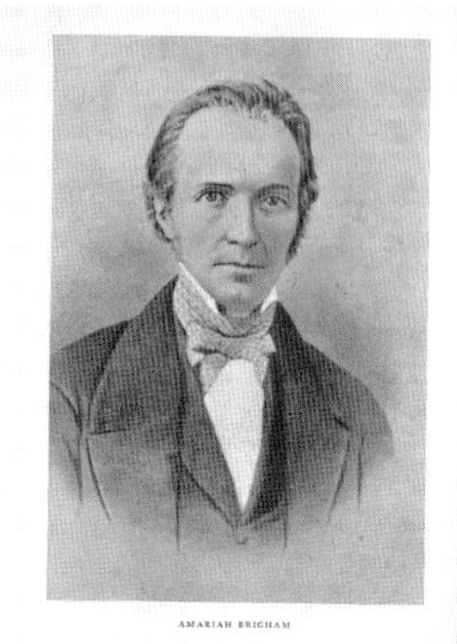

Official portrait of Dr. Amariah Brigham. *Oneida County History Center.*

physician and was successful for many years in the United States and abroad. He would marry and had four children, with his only son dying at the age of twelve in 1848 from a dysentery outbreak in Utica. Dr. Brigham served as the superintendent for the Retreat of the Insane in Hartford, Connecticut, before he received the assignment of running the New York State Lunatic Asylum at Utica. Dr. Brigham came to Utica to take over the largest and most expensive asylum ever built up to that point and the first of its kind in New York State. He opened the asylum in January 1843, when only the front part was finished, and it quickly filled. More room became a necessity He had the stressful work of overseeing structural changes and completions, hiring and training the staff, all the while pushing forth his innovative approach to patient care. Additional funds of $60,000 were acquired, and the two wings were completed by 1847, bringing the total cost up to that point to $448,980. In the first year of operation, Dr. Brigham welcomed 276 patients from 48 counties with the new wings able to host up to 500 patients.

That same year, Dr. Brigham brought on his assistant physician, Dr. H.A. Buttolph; Cyrus Chatfield, steward; Mrs. Chatfield, matron; Edmund A. Wetmore, treasurer; and staff to assist in the laundry, kitchen and other areas. The original staff numbered forty-one, and all took up residence at the asylum. In addition, staff members were banned from drinking alcohol or partaking in tobacco. Dr. Brigham admired Dr. Philippe Pinel, a leader of mental illness treatment who took patients out of dungeons and chains. Pinel was of the opinion that mental illness was a disease. At that time, many thought it was possession or the devil taking hold. There would be no dungeons or chains under Dr. Brigham's tenure, and he used reinforced rooms for violent and noisy patients, along with leather or cloth mittens, leather muffs and wristbands. This civil and humane treatment was much different than at the poorhouses, almshouses and jails in which they had been hidden away. When violent patients arrived at the asylum bound in chains, Dr. Brigham would have them taken off right then and there. He put them to work in fresh air with occupational purpose. In stark contrast, Dr. Brigham invented the Utica crib, which was like a baby crib but adult

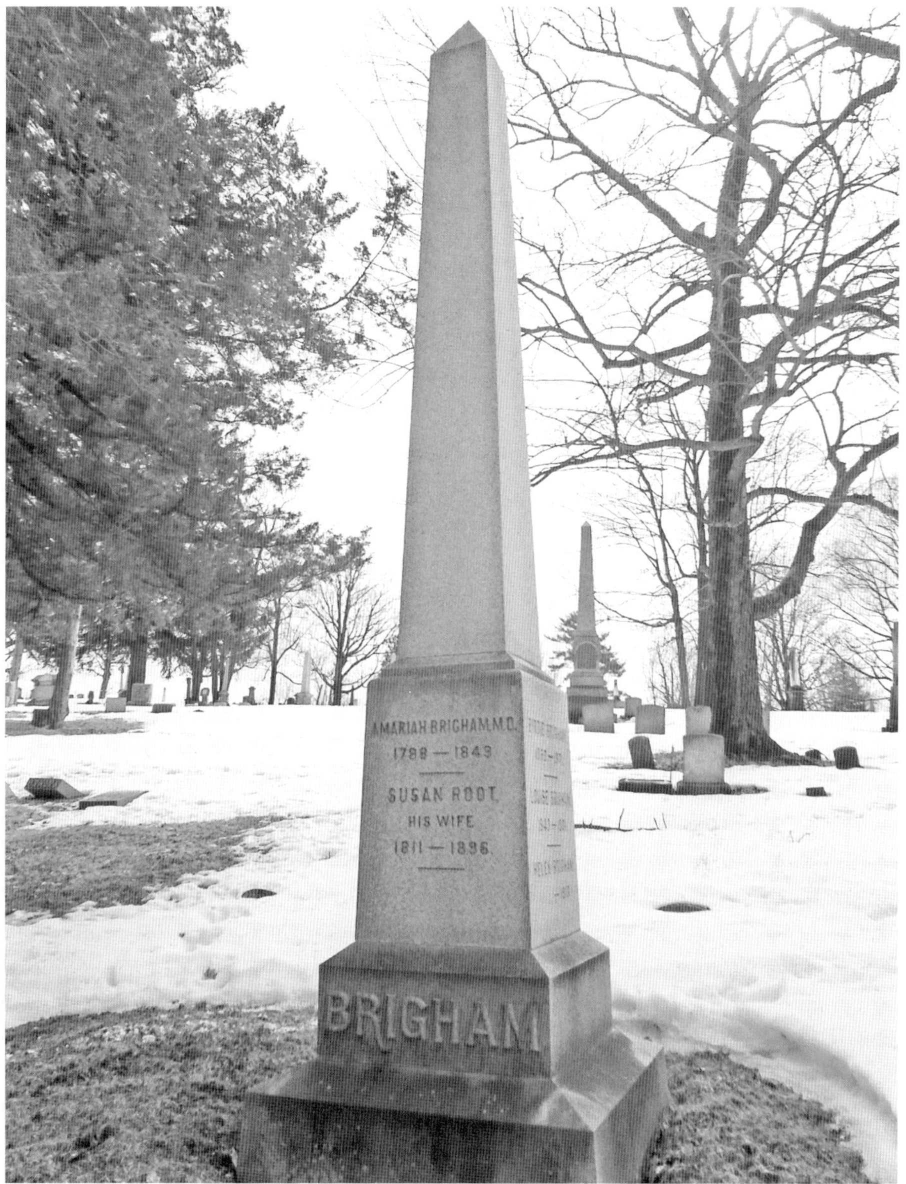

Dr. Amariah Brigham's grave at Forest Hill Cemetery at Utica, New York. *Courtesy Dennis Webster.*

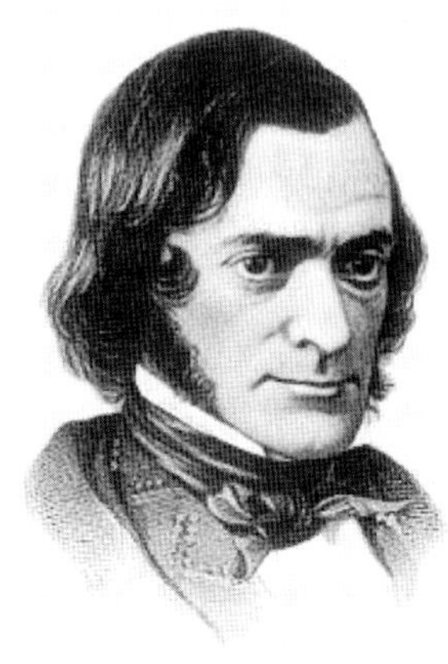

Andrew Jackson Downing designed the grounds of Old Main in the picturesque Gothic style. *Oneida County History Center.*

size with a lid that would lock down and hold the patient in place. This device became the most popular restraint in the world and would be in mass use for the next forty years.

Dr. Brigham was considered the leader in the "cult of curability" and considered "manual labor as the most essential as a curative means." He had patients in various occupations within and outside the asylum that he felt would cure or assist in their mental well-being. He also started the first fair at the asylum, where patient-made items would be for sale. This fair was January 1844 and featured needlework, carved dolls and wooden utensils. The fair was a huge success, based on the superior quality of the made items—so much so the New York State Fair came to Utica the next year and Dr. Brigham had a booth with the patient items on display and for sale. The quality of the goods won numerous awards for the patients. The *American Journal of Insanity* was created at the asylum and boomed to national sales and is still published today as the *American Journal of Psychiatry*. Dr. Brigham was a prolific writer and published many books on the anatomy of the brain and mental treatment. He also kept a huge number of books on mental illness in a large library that was turned over to the asylum after his death.

Dr. Brigham was highly respected nationally and testified at the trial of a Black man, William Freeman, who was accused of murdering four people in Auburn, New York, on March 12, 1846. Brigham would be thrust in a powerful trial that pitted the then state attorney general John Van Buren, son of President Van Buren, on the side of the prosecution with William A. Seward for the defense. The community wanted a public hanging, which was common for murderers of the time. It wouldn't be until later in the century that hangings were replaced with the electric chair—at Auburn, of all places. Freeman had just been released after serving five years in state prison when he was accused of committing murder. The defense called Dr. Brigham to testify to bolster its claim that William Freeman was a lunatic and thus deserved to be committed to an asylum and not put to death. The prosecution jumped when Dr. Brigham declared he could diagnose insanity just by looking at a person. The prosecuting lawyers made the audience abuzz when they asked Dr. Brigham to scan the crowd and point

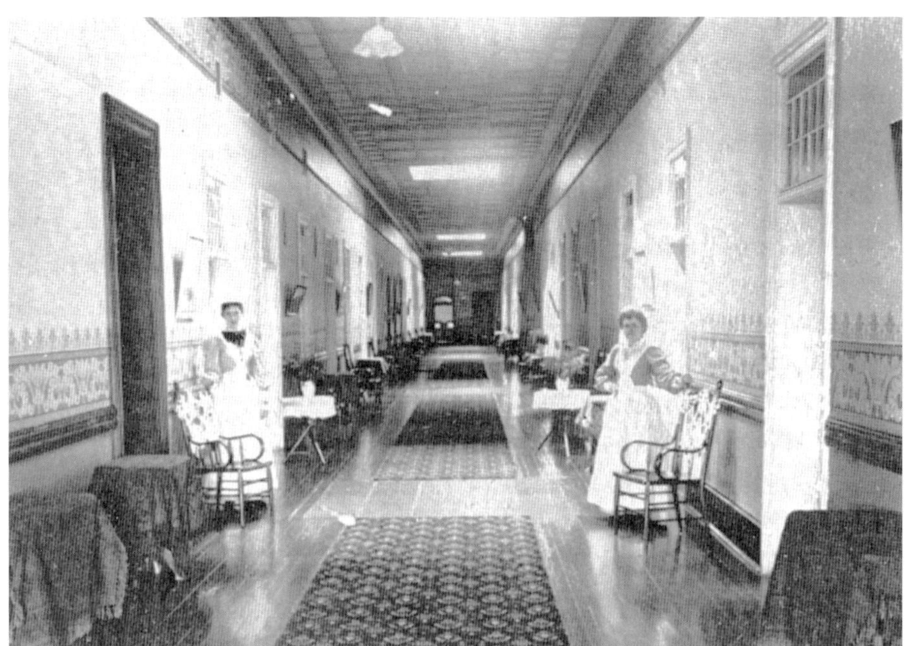

Matrons in the halls inside Old Main. *New York State Archives*.

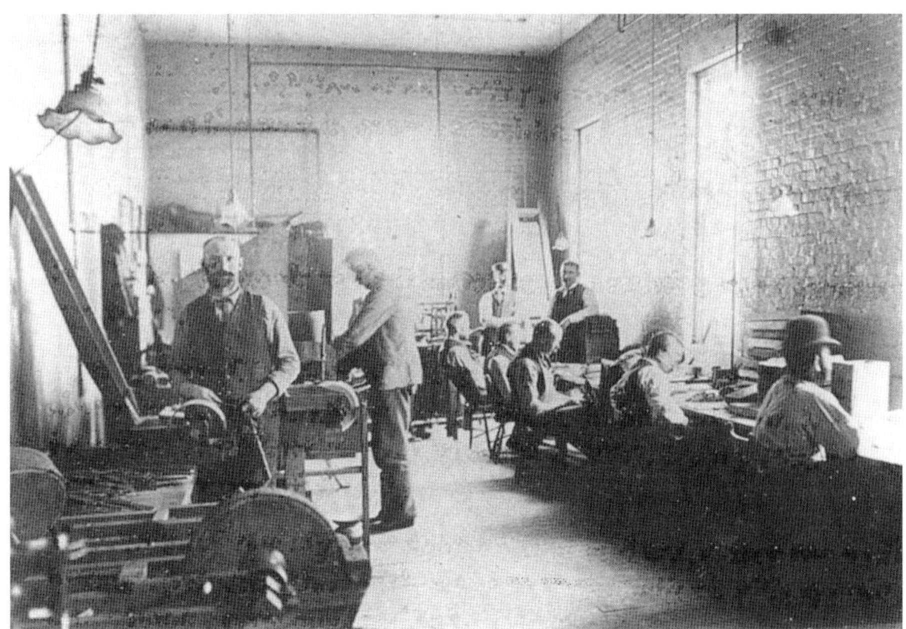

Patients on their job at the asylum workshop. *New York State Archives*.

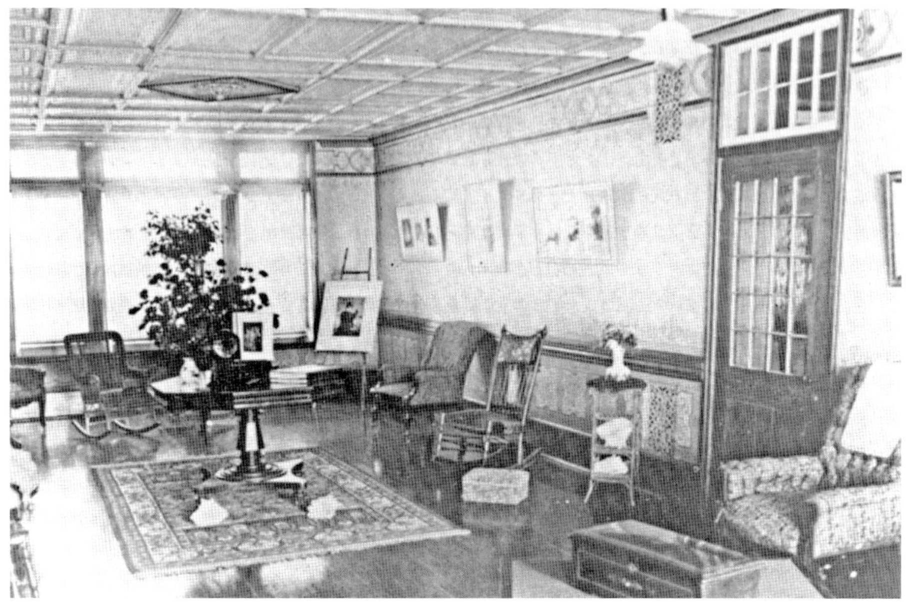

Lounge where patients could relax. *New York State Archives.*

out anybody who might be insane. He scanned the room with what was described as a "piercing brilliant gaze" as he looked into the eyes of each person. Dr. Brigham came upon a stable hand who had wandered into the courtroom, pointed at the man and declared, "Here is your insane man." The crowd erupted, and the man jumped up and had to be restrained by officers, who cleared him from the courtroom. This made the crowd come to Dr. Brigham's side, and his testimony kept Freeman from hanging, although the man was declared guilty of murder in the first degree and spent his life in jail. This incident has gone down as one of the most dramatic courtroom scenes in history.

Dr. Brigham has been described as a difficult, stubborn, opinionated man, yet he was also a tireless advocate and worker who wanted to not only cure mental illness but prevent it as well. He helped usher in a new psychology in America and inspired many to take his theories further and improve them. The number of patients swelled under the leadership of Dr. Brigham. In 1847, the Lunatic Asylum was the largest in the United States, with 380 single rooms for the insane, 24 for their caregivers, 20 dormitories that could accommodate 5 to 12 persons each, 16 day rooms, 12 dining rooms and 24 bathing rooms, with the same number of water closets and clothing closets. A gas system of lighting was added at an additional cost of $5,000.

Adding to the stress on Dr. Brigham was the legislature, which passed a law allowing the transfer of the criminally insane to the asylum. Homicidal maniacs would bring all sorts of challenges for the staff and stresses on the current patients. All counties but three in New York State sent lunatics to the asylum. In 1848, overcrowding became a reality; there were 877 patients in the asylum that year. In his last report on the asylum in 1848, Dr. Brigham listed 2,014 patients admitted since the opening. All were not charged to the public; some had paid by their own means or by family or friends. These private-pay patients paid from $2.50 to $4.00 per week, while New York State paid $2.00 per week for the indigent. Brigham was fiscally responsible and said to have had "Yankee thrift," along with his trusted treasurer, Edmund Wetmore. After a short illness, Dr. Amariah Brigham died at the age of fifty-one on September 9, 1849. His remains are buried in the grand and historic Forest Hill Cemetery in Utica, New York.

Moral Treatment by Dr. Brigham

Dr. Brigham was a leader in the field of "moral treatment" and put his theory to the test when he became the first superintendent of the New York State Lunatic Asylum at Utica. Dr. Brigham put forward his opinion in an extensive article in the *American Journal of Insanity*. He had started this progressive medical journal right in Utica at the asylum building. In the article, he states that when an insane person is removed from the home, they should be treated with respect and dignity. They would be placed in an asylum that would teach self-control through manual labor, a strict regimen of life to distract the mind from morbid thoughts. There would be mandatory religious services on Sundays, occupations and a range of activities essential to moral treatment of the insane.

The moral treatment was also a deciding factor in setting up the Lunatic Asylum at Utica. Dining halls, lounges, rooms and workshops would all look like patients' homes or places of employment. They would no longer wear ragged, dirty clothing; instead, asylum residents would don matching, clean clothing that would be washed and pressed regularly. The attendants, nurses and other staff would wear neat, clean uniforms to be professional. When visitors, families or dignitaries walked the hallways of Old Main, they were pleased to see the patients in a clean, well-run facility.

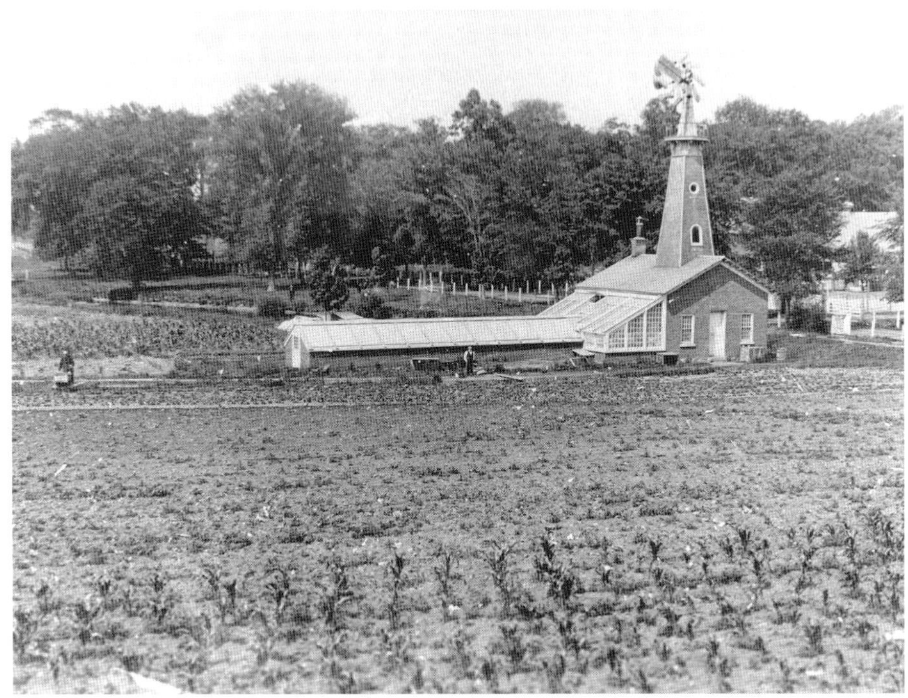

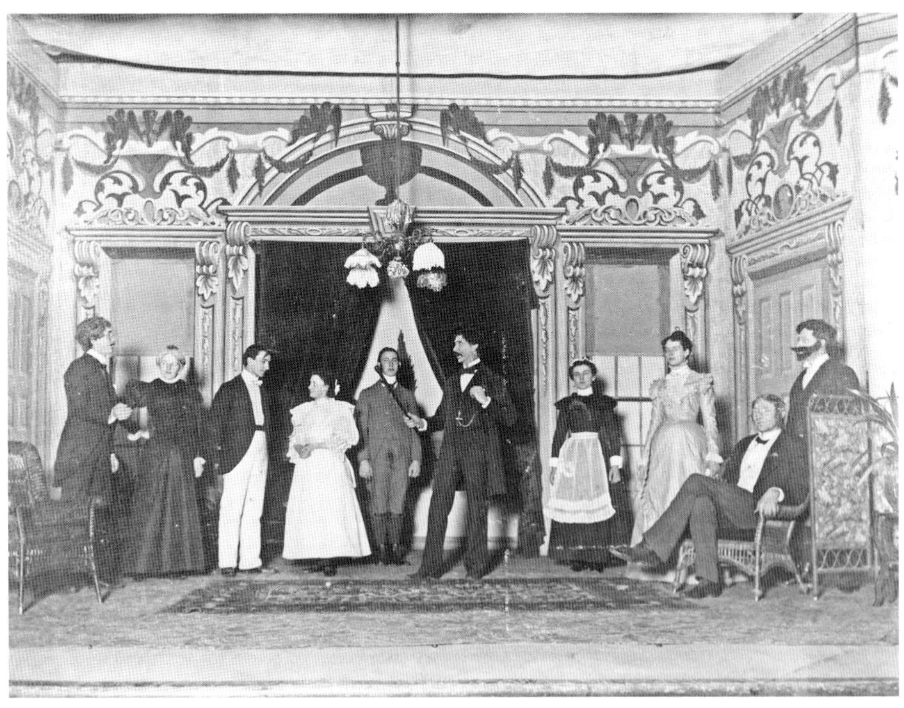

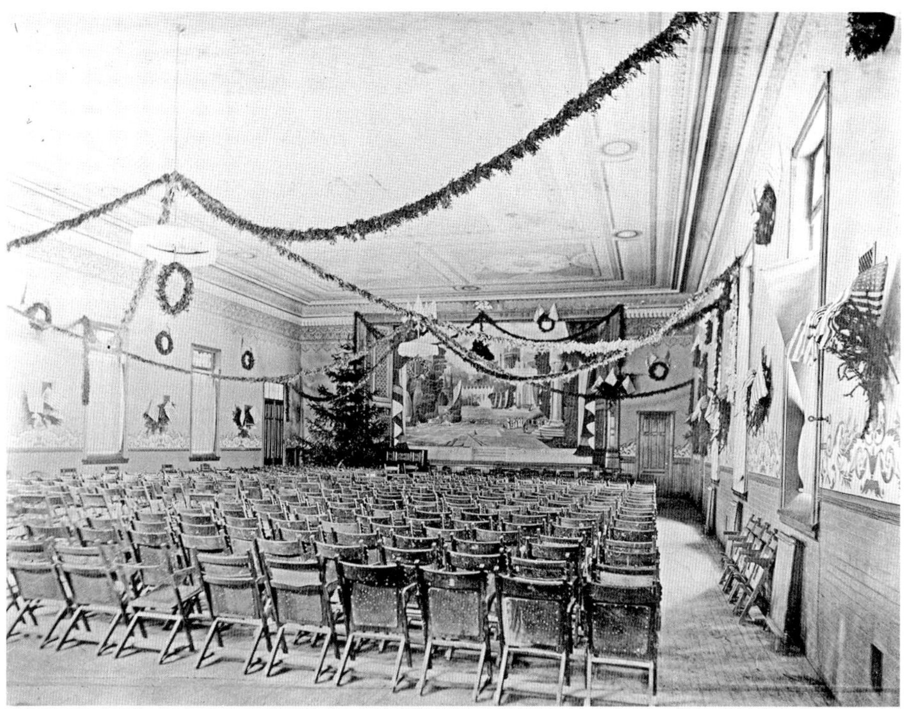

Opposite, top: The Utica State Hospital farm provided work for the patients and food for their table. *New York State Archives.*

Opposite, bottom: Patients of the asylum putting on a play for fellow patients and staff. *New York State Archives.*

Above: Asylum stage where minstrel shows, plays and the asylum band played. *Oneida County History Center.*

In his writing, Dr. Brigham mentioned Pinel treating patients with kindness but some places in the world still treating the insane quite brutally. He acknowledged the belief of lunacy being handed down by the devil but asserted that the better treatment of the insane had to do with an increase in knowledge. He said ignorance had caused the insane to be persecuted, mistreated and put to death in the past. The patients of the modern nineteenth-century asylum were not witches, heretics or devils; they were human beings with diseases that are sometimes difficult to diagnose. The spread of science helped to end heretic diagnosis.

Dr. Brigham called Pinel bold and brave for unchaining fifty maniacs at the Bicetre Hospital in France in 1792. Pinel made this move after vast learning and research into the insane. He tried his moral treatment system for several years before publishing it to the world. The system would be adapted and changed as it progressed to England then America. Dr. Brigham added elements such as occupations and activities. Giving the mentally ill tasks like cooking, cleaning, working in the print shop, sewing, making and repairing shoes and dozens of other jobs in the asylum kept the mind fresh and occupied. This was revolutionary at the time and made the Lunatic Asylum at Utica one of the most popular places to visit in the United States.

Dr. Brigham gives credit to Dr. Benjamin Rush, who started the moral treatment movement in this country and was called, by Dr. Brigham, a man of great intelligence and benevolence. Dr. Brigham learned from Dr. Rush to treat the patients with dignity and look them in the eye. If you wish to obtain respect and obedience, you should never show levity to the patients. This would extend to the furnishings of the asylum, the food served and the work doled out to the patients. The law of kindness applied.

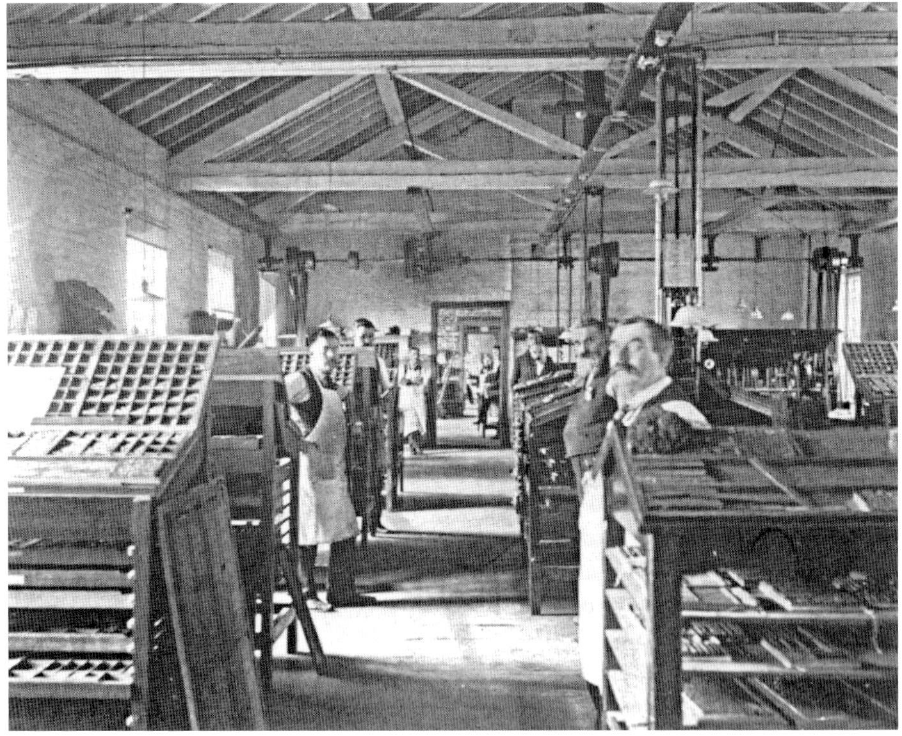

Print shop where patients worked. *New York State Archives*.

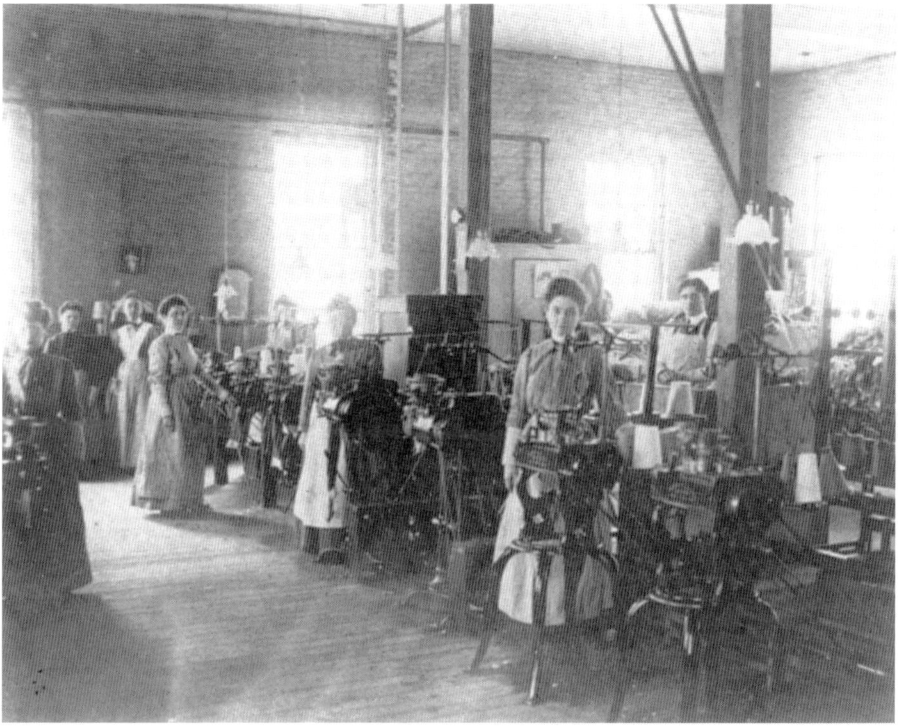

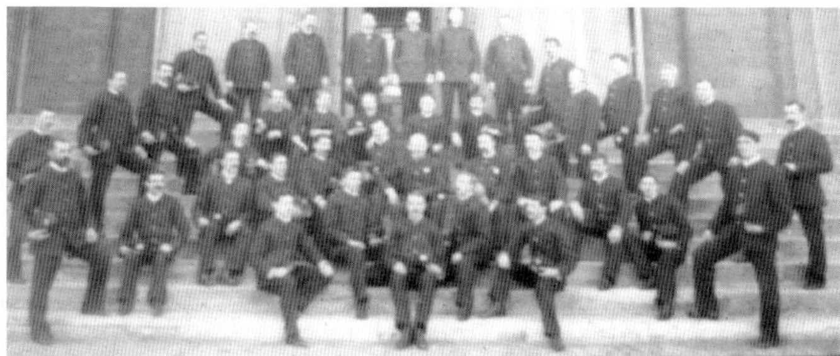

Above: Patients in the workshop. *New York State Archives.*

Left: Staff members posing on the front steps. *New York State Archives.*

Dr. Brigham felt that the moral treatment had neither been updated nor improved since Pinel, and the Lunatic Asylum at Utica would have a few changes. One would be that not all patients were to be treated with medicine and potions and that bodily labor and outdoor exercise for fresh air would be mandatory. Reading, acting in plays, music and drama would all be added as a way to keep the mind occupied and busy. At the time, these were radical and new ways of treating the insane. Dr. Brigham felt the moral treatment was more important than the medicine when treating the insane.

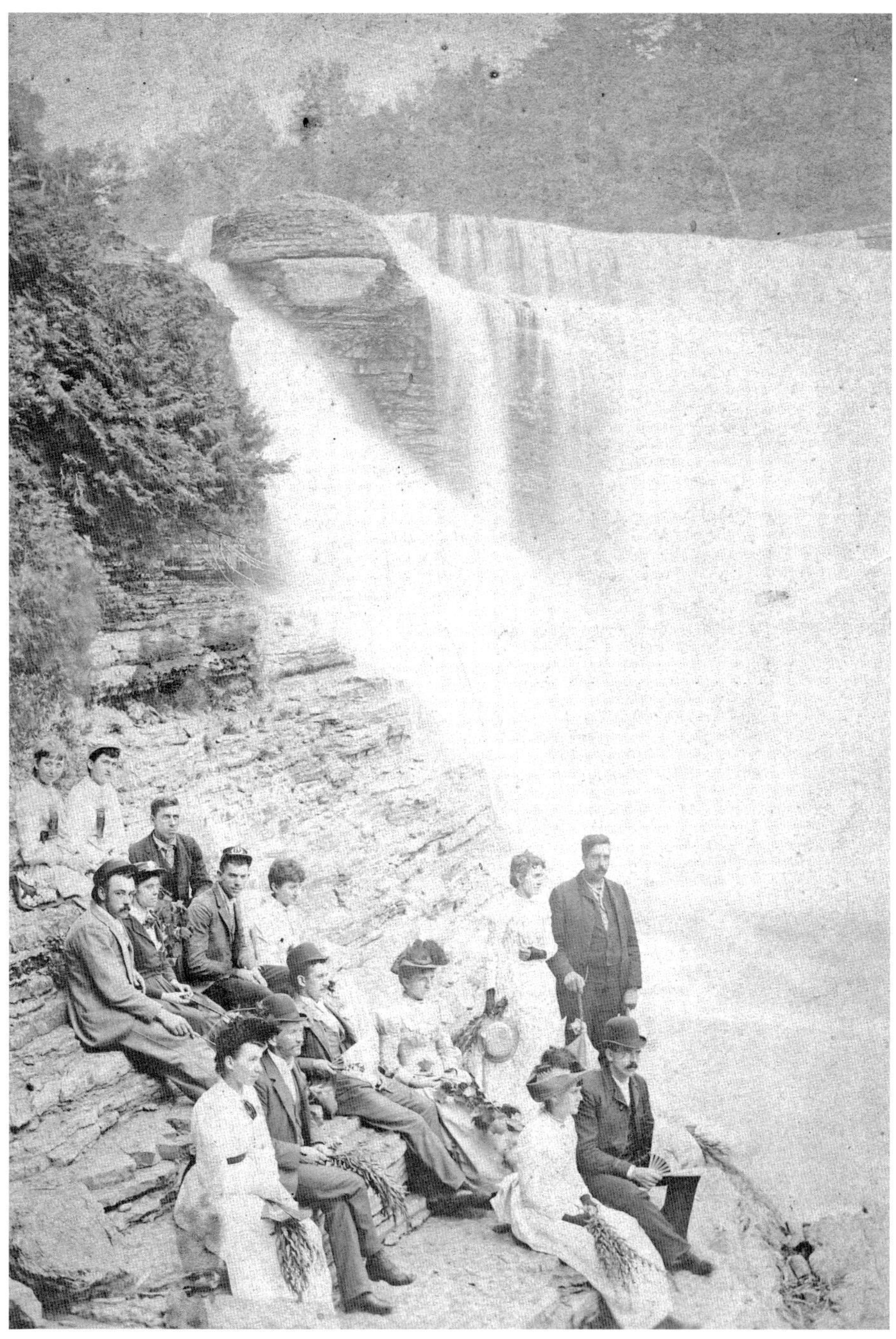

Patients visiting Trenton Falls, New York, on August 4, 1890. *Courtesy Dennis Webster.*

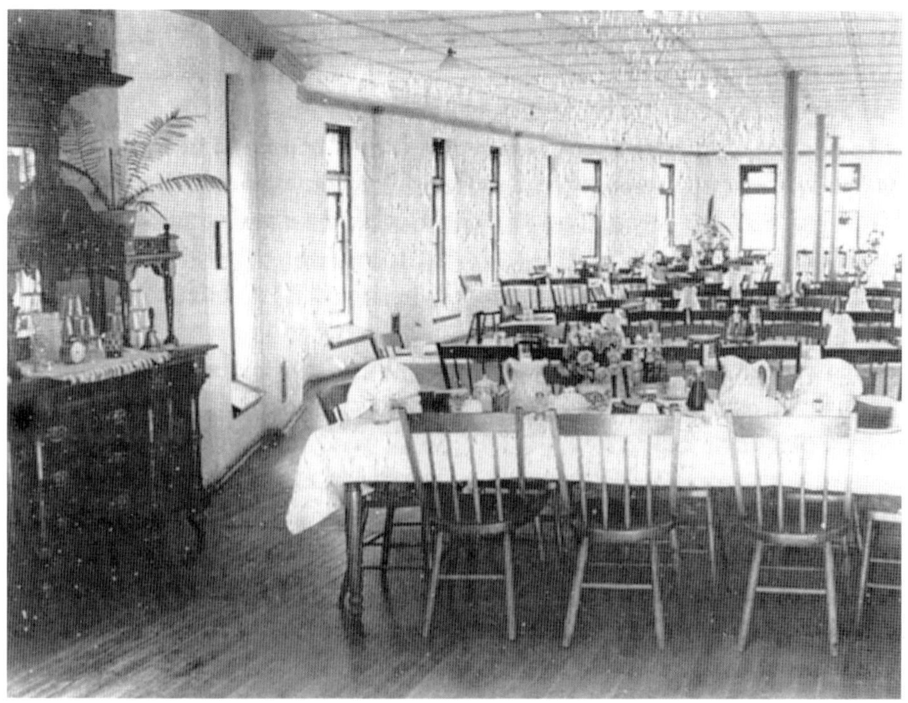

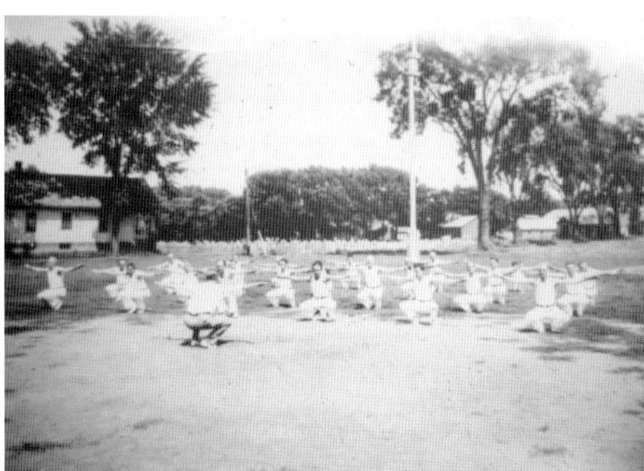

Above: The lavish dining hall where patients ate their meals. *New York State Archives*.

Left: Exercise and fresh air were part of the therapy. *New York State Archives*.

Dr. Brigham felt that engaging the brain in successful outcomes and new ways of thinking would be beneficial and healthy to the patient. Working on the asylum farm, working in their occupations in the facility and partaking in the arts were all ways of assisting in the care of the lunatic. At the time, other asylums in Europe were using manual labor but only for those most insane and incurable. Dr. Brigham felt those capable of being cured could benefit greatly from the work. This is what set Old Main's moral treatment apart from all others. He felt that asylums should be well stocked with books, maps, apparatus of sciences and collections of natural history. Dr. Brigham wanted all patients to engage in reading, writing, drawing, music, arithmetic, geography, history and other subjects. It's easy for us today to look at this moral treatment and say that it is natural and the right thing to do. It was revolutionary, brave and a huge leap in treatment of those with mental illness back in 1843 when Old Main opened its doors. Dr. Brigham deserves to be revered for championing the diagnosis and treatment of those who have mental illness.

Old Main Leadership on Opening in 1843

Board of Managers

Honorable T.H. Hubbard, Utica, president
Nicholas Devereux, Esq., Utica
C.B. Coventry, MD, Utica
A. Munson, Esq., Utica
C.A. Mann, Esq., Utica
Honorable J. Sutherland, Geneva
Hon D. Buel Jr., Troy
T.R. Beck, MD, Albany
A.V. Williams, MD, New York

Resident Officers

A. Brigham, MD, superintendent and physician
H.A. Buttolph, MD, assistant physician
Cyrus Chatfield, steward
Mrs. Chatfield, matron
Edmund A. Wetmore, treasurer and secretary to the Board of Managers

Why would the term *lunatic* be used to describe patients and *Lunatic Asylum* for the structure to house the mentally ill in 1843? Because it was considered the proper phrasing at the time for those with mental illness. In time, the term *mentally retarded* would be used. This phrasing would ultimately be considered offensive, so in our modern age, *mentally disabled* is deemed the proper phrase. The Lunatic Asylum was a catch-all when it first opened and hosted children to senior citizens with everything from blindness, senility, mental disability, Tourette's and Alzheimer's, along with homicidal criminal maniacs. If you were poor and confused, you were placed in the asylum. It wouldn't be until a decade later that homicidal maniacs were moved to Auburn. At the time, this seemed humane and just. The word *lunatic* was the proper term for those considered insane in the mid-nineteenth century. The word comes from Middle English, *lunatic*; Old French, *lunatique*; and Latin, *luna*. This term for the mentally ill is attributed to the Roman historian Pliny the Elder and his "moist brain" theory and Greek philosopher Aristotle, who had theories about the phases of the moon affecting the mental state of humans.

American Phrenological Journal (1847)

Phrenology was the study of pointing out the relationship between the organ of the brain and the manifestations of the mind. Back in the early to mid-nineteenth century, phrenology was popular among those who studied mental health and insanity. The doctrine of phrenology stated that certain areas of the brain had certain operations like anger, fear, jealousy, hate, love and many more emotions. It was thought that the brain, being one large organ, could not deliver multiple functions or emotions at a time, so it had to be segmented into different operations that dealt with emotions and body functions. Phrenology says that if we had one functioning brain you could not walk and talk at the same time. The theory also stated that if mental derangement was caused by a brain disorder then the mind is insane or sane; however, the theory of phrenology is proven in lunacy, as some derangements are in only certain areas of the mind or functions while others are perfectly sane. This theory led to doctors stating that certain shapes of heads, eye placement, skull measurements and ear placement could determine lunacy or idiocy. Though eventually scientifically proven wrong, phrenology was an important advancement in treatment of those with mental illness. Science had started to come into play instead of blaming insanity on the movements of the moon or maneuvers by the

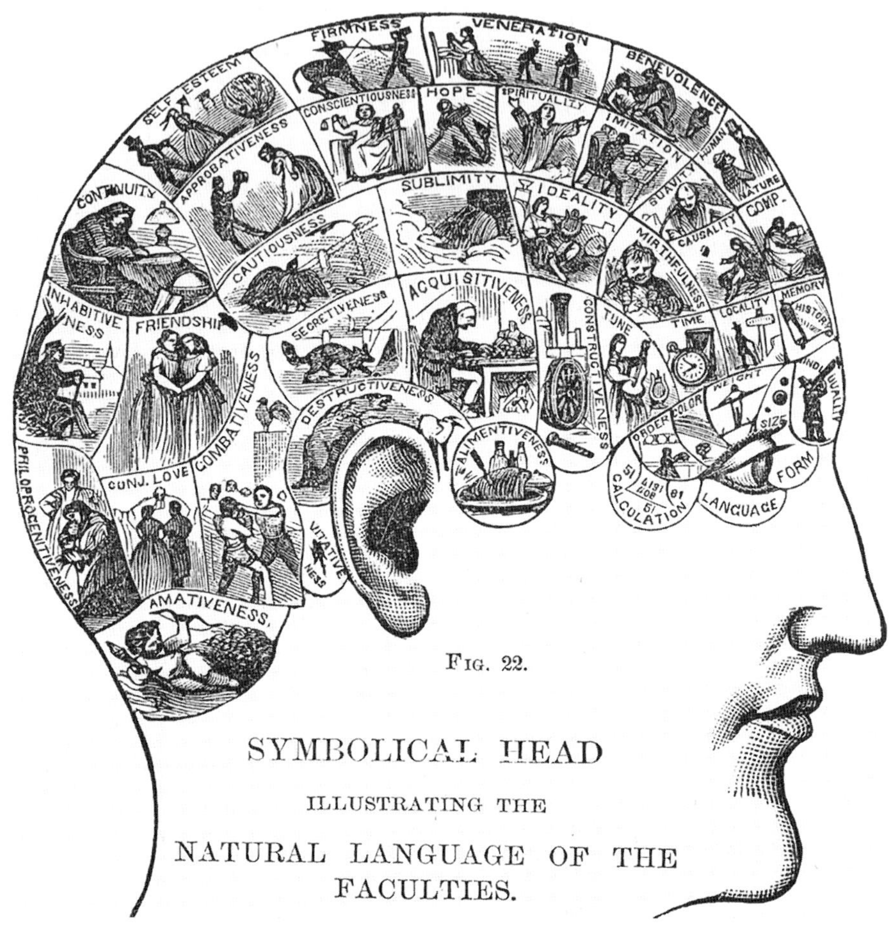

Diagram of phrenology brain with localized functions. *Courtesy Utica Public Library.*

devil. Scientific research and better patient care drove Old Main to be a worldwide leader in academic journals and research.

Architecture

The grand structure of Old Main was built in the Greek Revival style using hammered limestone from quarries in Little Falls and Stittville. The stones were carried to the asylum from Stittville using horse and carriage and from Little Falls by boat through the Erie Canal and the Chenango

Canal. Captain William Clarke was the architect of the Lunatic Asylum at Utica with the iconic grand Doric pillars welcoming visitors, staff and patients. The iconic six Doric pillars on the front of Old Main are 48 feet in height and 8 feet in diameter. The front main building is 550 feet in length and 50 foot in depth. In his book *Architecture: Nineteenth and Twentieth Centuries*, architectural historian Henry Russell Hitchcock wrote the following about Old Main: "No European public edifice has a grander Greek Doric portico than that which dominates the tremendous four story front block."

The original plans called for four wings forming a square with a courtyard in the middle. This design would accommodate one thousand patients, yet lack of funds would allow only the front and side wings to be built. In 1838, of the $50,000 appropriated by New York State for the structure, $46,000 had been spent on just the foundations. In May 1840, another $75,000 was appropriated to complete the main front and the two wings. The extra foundation stones that were to be the last back wing were used to construct a carriage house that eventually became the garage. More appropriations brought the cost up to $285,000. In April 1842, another $16,000 was given

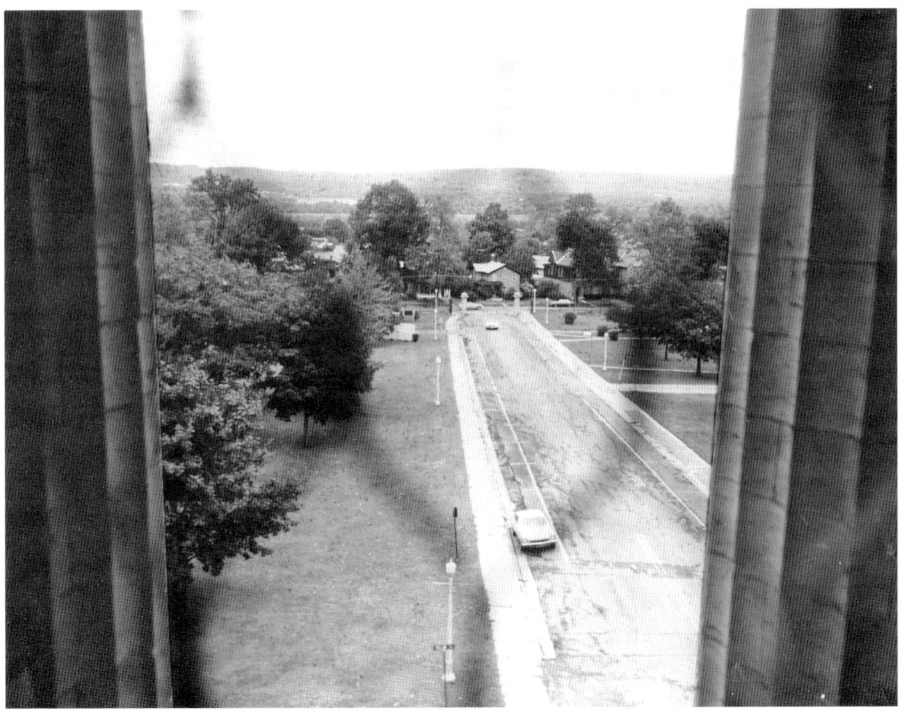

View through the pillars. *New York State Archives.*

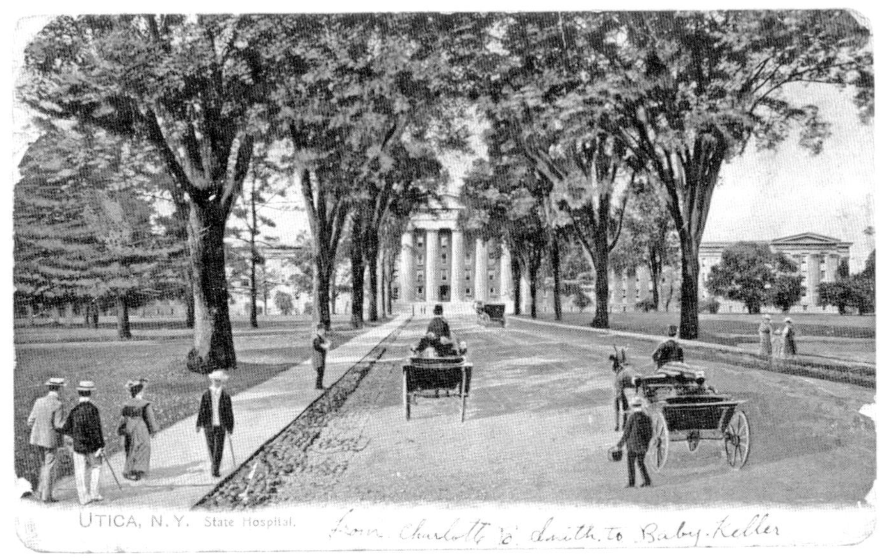

Postcard sent from Old Main to a loved one. *Courtesy Dennis Webster.*

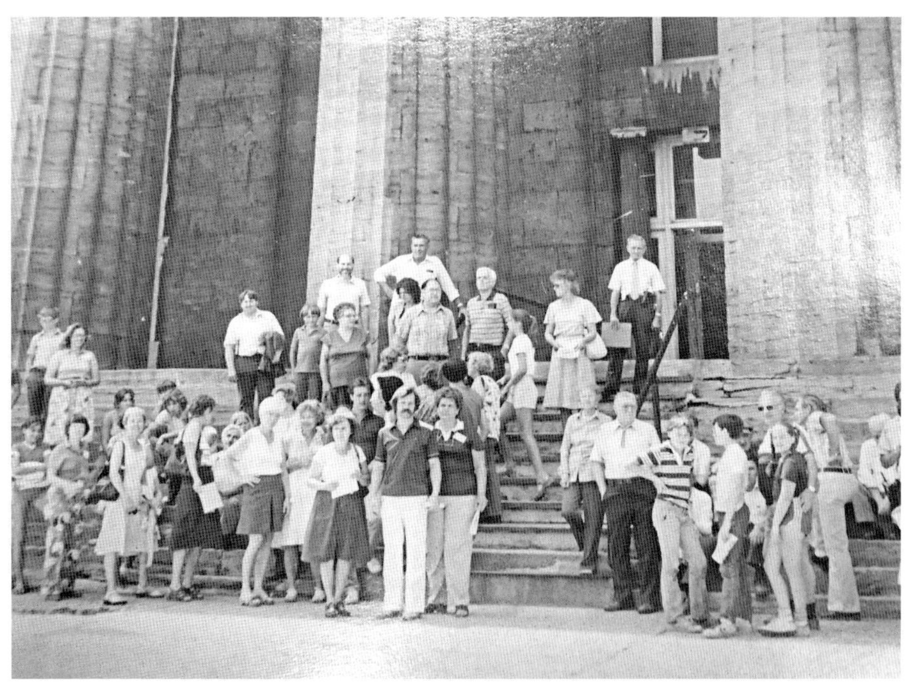

Old Main attracts visitors. *New York State Archives.*

by the New York State legislature to furnish the asylum with a water supply, a drainage system and other necessities. Water would be served by large wells on the property. The illumination at night would be provided by oil lamps. The heating would be provided by the most advanced wood-burning furnaces at the time, which used two cords of wood per day. Several were installed to give heat to the largest parts of the asylum.

The asylum opened with 380 single rooms, 24 housed attendants, 20 dorm rooms that held up to 12 patients, 16 parlors, 12 dining rooms, 24 bathing rooms, 24 closets and 24 water closets. Andrew Jackson Downing designed the lavish gardens and landscaping in the picturesque Gothic style. He has been called the father of American landscape architecture. The grounds included one thousand planted trees, hundreds of shrubs and a greenhouse loaded with hundreds of flower and plant species. For most of the nineteenth century, a tall wooden fence surrounded Old Main, but it was not meant to keep the patients inside. It was to keep deer and other animals from eating the fruits and vegetables as well as to keep young men and boys from approaching and harassing the young lady patients. The Old Main building was placed in the National Register of Historical Places on October 26, 1971.

Rules, Regulations and Bylaws

The following is a summary of the *Rules, Regulations and By-Laws of the New York State Lunatic Asylum*, published in 1842 then revised in 1853. The book states that patients are "inmates" and that they are to be taken care with the "Law of Kindness." People employed at the Lunatic Asylum were told that their duty was to increase happiness and ease suffering. The bylaws state: "We are dealing with fellow creatures, who deprived of reason, are not responsible for their conduct." The regulations attest that patients are violent and led astray by perverted senses. The employees are told they cannot return harsh words, neglect the lunatics, treat them unkindly or return any kind of violence. Employees are mandated to not be cold, insensitive or negligent but offer their best care.

The Lunatic Asylum was put under the overall governance of a board of managers that consisted of the president of the board, an auditing committee to watch spending, a treasurer, a secretary and at-large members. They were required to have their annual board meeting with all members in attendance and quarterly meetings with a majority on hand. They were also mandated to visit randomly. All members of the board were banned from doing any business with the asylum, receiving a gratuity from any lunatic or accepting gifts from any family member or friend of a patient.

The publication introductory pages summarize why the Lunatic Asylum was built and its purpose. In keeping in the flavor of the time and context, here is the exact wording:

> *This Asylum has been erected, at great expense, by the State, that the insane may have a safe retreat, in the care of those who have learned the true mode of managing them; in whose hands they may be rescued from the cruelties and coercions which they generally meet with in this world; and where, under the benign restraints which kindness and benevolence impose, they may have every chance of recovery.*
>
> *The very first impulses of insanity are met at home and amongst friends, by resistance and opposition, from those who before yielded willing obedience to requirements, or who have acquiesced with cheerfulness in every reasonable indulgence. The apparent difference in the conduct of feelings of their friends, excites collision, arouses the passions, and awakes the prejudices of the victim of delusion. They now feel that the friends whom they loved and enjoyed have turned against them; that they purposefully thwart all their plans, oppose all their desires, and resist what they conceive to be their own best efforts to promote the happiness of both. The insane resist all these with violence, and indulge in wrath and bitterness against them.*
>
> *For these reasons it becomes desirable that they should be removed to the care of strangers, whose efforts to make them comfortable, they often appreciate correctly and acknowledge gratefully. From strangers they will also submit to restraints without a murmur, which would excite the greatest hostility to friends.*
>
> *In this institution the duty now devolves upon us. In the various departments of business, and of care, we all have daily much to do with the inmates of the Asylum. Some of us devote our whole time to this duty. It becomes us all seriously to consider how this duty shall be performed; what discipline of feeling and what subjugation of temper there shall be with us, that we may ever administer the "LAW OF KINDNESS" to its full extent, and in its proper spirit.*
>
> *When we accept a place in this Asylum, we assume a responsibility which it should be our constant desire to fulfil to our own satisfaction and that of our employers; it should be performed conscientiously, so as*

to be approbated by our MAKER, who will be strict to mark injustice or oppression to unfortunate and suffering fellow men.

No individual is worthy of a place in such an institution who labors for wages only. Duty, a desire to improve the condition of all within the sphere of our influence, to increase the happiness and lesson the sufferings of each and all the inmates, should be the governing motive of our daily conduct. We must never forget that are dealing with fellow creatures who, being deprived of reason, are not responsible for their conduct. The regulating power of moral action is withheld from them; hence they are capricious, passionate, and often violent. They often also misjudge, and are led astray by perverted sense or by delusions of the understanding, which carry them far away from the properties of rational conduct. How exceedingly wicked and improper, therefore, to harbor a spirit of revenge, or to retaliate for injuries done us by such individuals!

It is because they are unable to control themselves, and because they will not readily acquiesce in the directions of their friends, that many of these individuals are placed in the Asylum. From us they are to have every comfort and every indulgence, which individually or collectively, will promote their best good. To us they look for sympathy and counsel, for assistance in their various troubles and perplexities. We should enter deeply into their feelings, and show our willingness to spend our time and strength to promote their happiness, and recovery to health.

If we withhold what they may reasonably require, we do them injustice, and violate our duty. If we treat them with neglect, or with unkind and hasty language; if in any way we tantalize them, or recriminate when they assail us with violent or abusive words, we may do them irreparable injury, for which we all ought to feel, and certainly shall be held responsible

Persuasion with a proper spirit, will generally be followed by a quiet acquiescence in all reasonable requirements. Much depends upon the MANNER of our intercourses with the insane. We should never be cold and insensible to their wants, never hasty and impatient in our intercourse, never turn a deaf ear to their representations, never treat them with neglect, nor with feelings of superiority, but mingle with them in kindness, address them with respect and affection, and we shall secure their confidence, and gain their affections, both of which are necessary to their management.

Resident officers included a superintendent, whose job it was to oversee the day-to-day operations of the Lunatic Asylum, to hire and manage the employees and establish discipline in all departments. The first superintendent of the asylum was Dr. Amariah Brigham. He was directed by these rules to visit patients daily to learn their conditions, direct treatments and keep all patient records pertaining to home, age, sex, name, mental condition, and whether they were released as cured, died or eloped (ran away). Any time a member of the board requested it, the superintendent would have to produce patient records for examination. He would have to produce a summary report to the board annually and include any experiments, opinion, conditions and other factoids of the operation. Under the direction of the superintendent, there were a matron and a steward. The men and women were housed in separate wings, and only men and women provided direct patient care. The matron oversaw all the female employees and the steward all the men. These direct patient care employees were called attendants.

Assistant physicians were mandated to oversee the wards, the stewards, matrons, and all the attendants. They were to visit each ward once in the morning and once in the afternoon. They needed to write reports that describe patients who needed special attention, seclusion, restraint or removal. They were also to keep records of personality changes and treatments. They needed to be sure of the warmth and comfort of the patients and supervise their bathing. They must attend to all visitors and attend to correspondence with friends and relatives of the lunatics. All of this was part of their jobs, plus anything assigned by the attending physician.

The treasurer was mandated to keep all books, track all invoices, record all vouchers and produce meticulous records of all financial transactions and must produce them on demand by the board or the asylum superintendent.

The steward was in charge of all male patients and attendants. He could hire and fire attendants and had to be sure all patients and staff were in their beds at the ringing of the night bell. He was to be sure all arose at the ringing of the morning bell and must report any abuse immediately to the superintendent. He must watch the shops, the farms, the rooms, the apartments and outbuildings are kept in good order. He must ensure all rules were being followed and the orders of the superintendent carried out.

The matron was in charge of all female patients, ensuring they were well treated, well fed, kindly taken care of by the nurses and that their bedding was clean and the rooms well ventilated. She was to supervise the sewing room and be sure every patient garment was marked with the name of the patient. She was to see that all who were sick were treated well and to follow the orders of the superintendent. They must report any negligence or misconduct by staff toward the lunatics. She also supervised the kitchen, where mostly patients would prepare and cook the food.

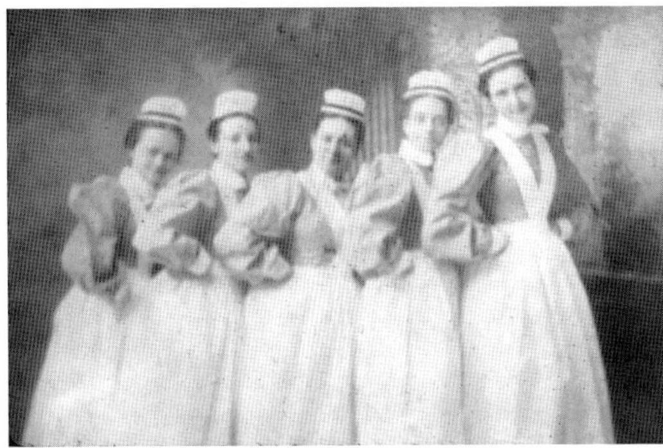

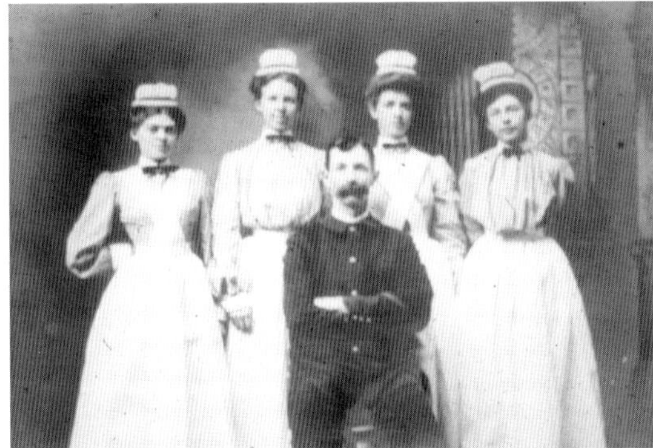

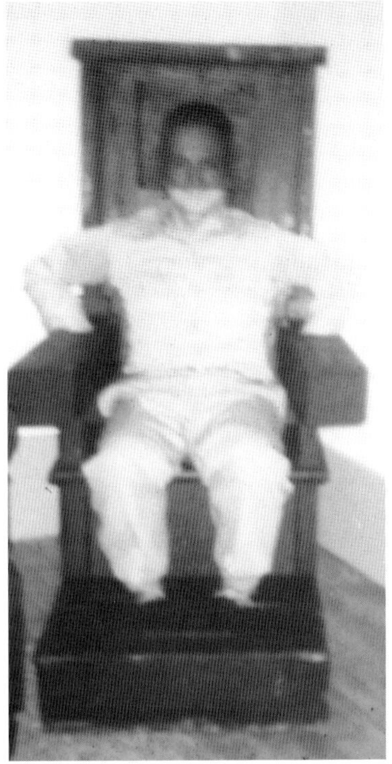

Left, top: Matrons posing in their uniforms. *New York State Archives.*

Left, bottom: Staff picture showing work uniforms. *New York State Archives.*

Right: Demonstration of a nineteenth-century patient-restraining device. *New York State Archives.*

Apothecaries were always on staff and had to be physicians, medical students or druggists. They must live at the asylum. They must administer all medicine as prescribed by the doctors and keep records of the medicinal applications. They could not leave the apothecary shop without permission. They must provide moral influence on the patients. The steward's assistant must visit the kitchen every morning, the bakery and the washroom and inspect their condition and report this to the steward. He must perform all duties assigned by the steward and report to the superintendent any instances of unfaithfulness, inefficiency or misconduct. The matron's assistant was to remain in the office of the matron and attend to the reception and discharge of lunatics. When asked, she must also attend to visitors. She must be able to assist, when needed, in the kitchens, labor departments and supervision. Clerks received patient clothing when they were admitted and must ensure the personal clothing was clearly marked with the name of the owner and placed in the ledger book. They would deliver small items and jewelry to the steward for safekeeping.

Supervisors were assigned to the men's and women's wings—one each for rooms 1, 2, 3, 4 and 5; one for rooms 6, 7, 8 and 9; and one for rooms 10, 11 and 12. Each room would have twenty patients placed in them, with the most severe in room number 12. The supervisors were to report to the matron or steward all conditions and keep an eye on the care of those under their charge. Most importantly, they were to take care of new lunatics and be sure they were acclimated to the asylum and trained in their new duties. They were to be sure furniture was on hand and everyone attended religious services.

Overseers were employees who watched the bakery and the kitchen. They were to keep track of inventory and be sure there was safe use of all kitchen implements. They were to stop any rude or bad behavior in the bakery and kitchen and be sure there was no swearing or quarreling. They must ensure cleanliness and all food supplies are in good order. Food was owned by the state and must be used in a proper manner—not wasted or stolen. There were overseers of the washing and ironing rooms. They reported to the steward and matron and must ensure all garments brought to them were washed, ironed, sorted by their marks and returned neat and clean. No patients or visitors were allowed in the washing and ironing rooms unless approved by the superintendent. An engineer was to be on hand to oversee all engines, the boiler house, all machines in workshops, all equipment for fighting fires, sewers, gas and water supply.

The gardener oversaw the greenhouse, gardens and all garden tools. The farmer oversaw all farm animals, including chickens, cows, plow horses and pigs and all farm tools. The carriage driver took care of the horses not used on the farm and all maintenance of the carriages. Night watchers were to patrol the asylum at night. There were to be two on the ladies' ward and two on the men's ward. Their shift was from 9:00 p.m. to 6:00 a.m. and their main function was to watch for fires and, second, to watch for elopement (escapes). They were to be sure no lunatics were running loose. They must be quiet and enter into no discussions during the night. They rang the bell in the morning to signal the start of the day. They must patrol with a light in lantern and must never deviate from this rule.

Attendants and assistants could not show bad care in their dealings with the inmates, must have self-respect, must not use profane language or play games and must do everything to portray a positive influence. They were not allowed to use tobacco or alcohol. They must greet all patients with "good morning" or "good evening." They could not become violent with the lunatics or engage in heated words with them. If hit by a patient, they were not to return the blows. Assistants and attendants could not call patients by nicknames but only their names with the prefix Mr., Mrs. or Miss. They were not to apply any restraining device without approval of one of the physicians. They must assist patients in their bathing, comb their hair, assist in them getting dressed and making their beds. They could never leave patients alone. They must assist in serving food at mealtime and be sure no patient walked away with knives or forks. They must be watchful of lunatics attempting suicide and be diligent to stop attempts. They must keep an eye on all patients in their work plus outside in their work. They must not mock or make fun of patients.

No attendants or assistants were to leave the asylum without approval of the superintendent. All employees were under a one-year contract and had to sign a contract that if they did not give a one-month notice or were discharged for violating rules, they forfeited one month of pay. Chamber pots as well as spittoons must be cleaned daily. Soiled bedding should be taken to the washrooms immediately.

Time and duties were strict at the asylum. Bells were rung three times to signify when patients were to rise: 5:00 a.m. in May, June, July and August; 5:30 a.m. in April, September, October and November; 6:00 a.m. in December, January, February and March. Breakfast was placed on the tables and served at 6:30 a.m. during the summer; 7:00 a.m. in spring and fall; and 7:30 a.m. in the winter. Lunch was always served at 12:30 p.m. and dinner at 6:00 p.m. The asylum closed at 9:30 p.m. year-round. The Sabbath was closed to all work and visitors unless deemed necessary by the superintendent. All inmates and staff were to attend religious services unless illness or severe madness excused them. A chaplain was on hand to conduct all religious services.

Visitors were welcome and encouraged, as the asylum was constructed at a great expense to New York State taxpayers. Visitors were welcome Monday through Friday from 2:00 p.m. to 5:00 p.m., except holidays. All visitors must have admission tickets from the managers of the asylum and produce them upon request. The asylum managers reserved the right to refuse admission to visitors not deemed appropriate. Visitors must not ask for individual patient information unless a relative, then must refrain from discussing it in public. At the end of one year of satisfactory performance, each male employee may receive a gratuity of eight dollars and each female employee five dollars.

A lunatic could be sent to the asylum by an order from any court, judge, justice or a supreme court commissioner. The order or warrant copy must be presented upon admission to the superintendent. This warrant had to be signed by two physicians who certified the insanity of the person to be admitted. The person requesting a patient's admission would have to state Christian name, place of homestead and relationship to the lunatic, and the certification must be signed under oath. Each admitted lunatic must be clean, have a fresh haircut, must be free of vermin and any infectious contagious disease. Every admitted male lunatic was provided with two new shirts, a new and substantial coat, a vest, woolen cloth pantaloons, one pair of mittens or gloves, two pairs of wool stockings, a black stock or cravat, a good cap or hat, a new pair of boots or shoes, along with a comfortable outside garment. Each admitted female lunatic was given undergarments, shoes, stockings, a flannel petticoat, two dresses of good quality and a cloak or outside garment. The women were allowed to have better clothing for church services or outside travel in order to maintain their self-respect. All must be clearly marked and only worn when deemed for a useful purpose.

The Lunatic Asylum would admit those who were of the almshouse-variety mad but also those of wealth and prominence. The price of board for those committed by the county, which included washing, medicine and attendance, did not exceed $2.50 a week. Others of means were to pay $4.00 unless they made special arrangements with the management for extra attention or accommodations. Payments were to be made twice per year in the months of February and August. The counties that committed a patient had to pay at least the first six months of residence, even in the event of elopement or death. Upon death, the county that had committed the lunatic paid funeral expenses.

The act to create the New York State Lunatic Asylum at Utica was passed by the New York State Senate and Assembly on April 7, 1842. In this act, the board of managers were appointed and given all the rules and tasks to get the asylum built and staffed. It stated the chosen ones could be removed by the governor of New York State and future appointments to the board could be nominated by the governor but voted on and approved by the legislature. A majority of the board of managers had to live within a five-mile radius of the asylum. Salaries of officers were to be set by the board of managers, and the aggregate of the superintendent, assistant physician, treasurer, matron and steward was not to exceed $5,500. The clerk of Oneida County would hold the paperwork of the oath of office all officers swore upon hiring. The superintendent was the CEO and could fire any employee or officer but must submit cause in writing.

It was ingrained into the early days of the asylum to promote the Lord and a religious life for all the patients. Regular attendance of church services was mandatory for all patients and staff, with the services overseen by the Reverend Chauncey E. Goodrich. All except those confined to Utica cribs were to attend. If patients got out of control during church services, they would be removed and placed in a chair with wrist restraints. Most would behave and embraced the religious services that came with their being committed.

The Utica Crib

Dr. Brigham's moral treatment avoided the use of chains and chemical restraints. At the time, some chairs had restraints and straightjackets were also deployed, but these were not the rule at Old Main. Dr. Brigham tried to use religion, occupation, the arts and activities, yet there still remained some patients who were loud, disruptive and dangerous to the staff and fellow residents. Dr. Brigham had seen many kinds of restraining devices on his travels, especially in Europe. He did not like any of these devices, so he decided to invent his own. The Utica crib was like a baby's crib but long and

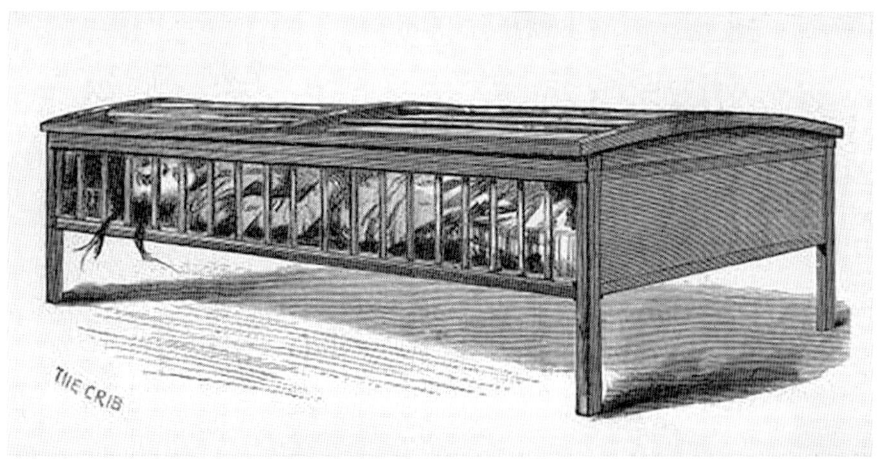

Artist rendering of Dr. Brigham's invention, the Utica crib. *Oneida County History Center.*

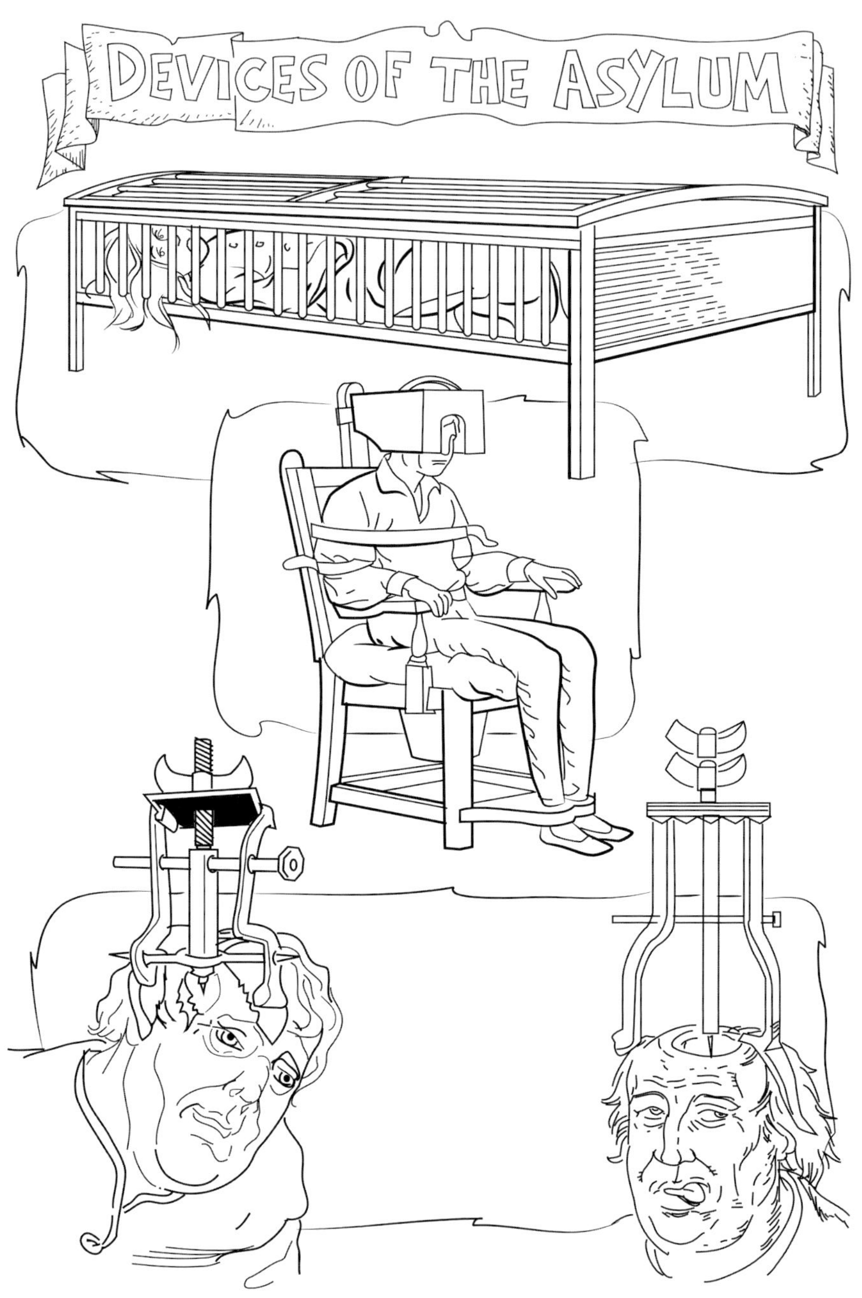

Nineteenth-century asylum devices for restraint. *By Luke McDonnell and Bill Anderson.*

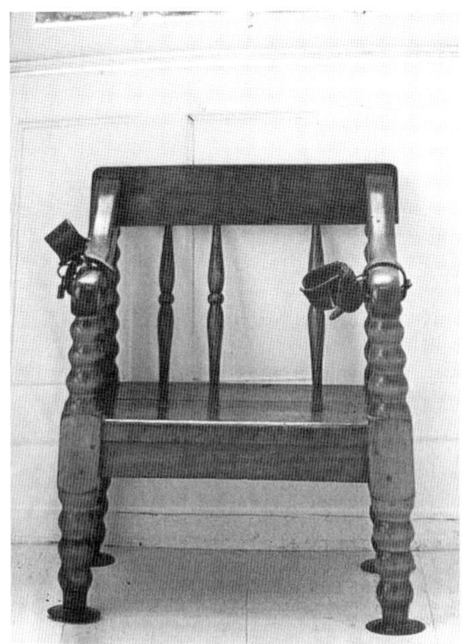

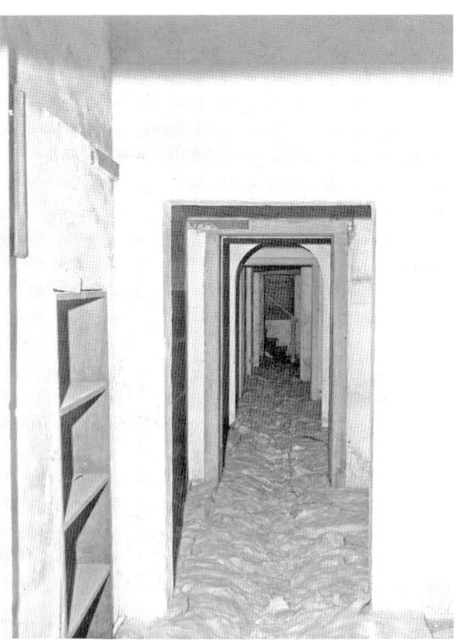

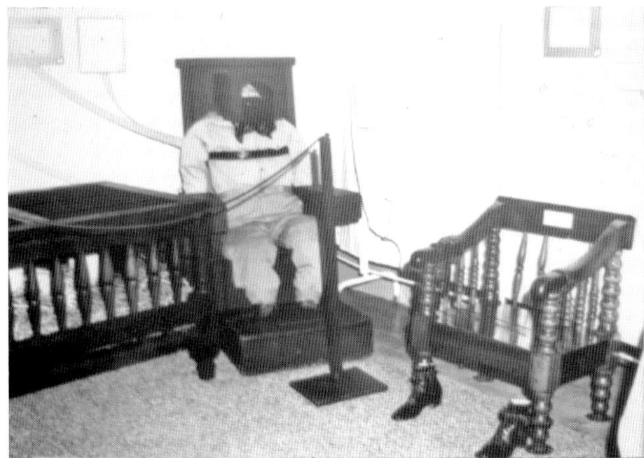

Above, left: Restraining chair on display in Old Main. *Courtesy Dennis Webster.*

Above, right: Basement of Old Main. *New York State Archives.*

Left: Restraining devices that were used for patients with manic symptoms. *New York State Archives.*

wide enough to accommodate an adult. There was a hinged lid that would lock. The depth was shallow, so an adult inside the Utica crib could not sit up or roll over. Open air could come in through the slats. When patients arrived at the asylum in chains, Dr. Brigham would have them removed as they entered the building. The Utica crib was used in extreme cases of mania.

The device became world famous and was used in every asylum in the civilized world. Eventually, the Utica crib fell out of favor and would not be used at the Lunatic Asylum in Utica after 1887. Moral treatment seems at odds to the use of a restraining device like the Utica crib. There were many who criticized the use of the Utica crib, but one of the harshest criticisms was that attendants at the asylum could place patients inside them, sometimes without the consent of the physicians. This was in conflict with the rule that had been set by the board of managers. The device was harshly criticized by Dr. William Hammond, an expert in mental health. He said in an article in the *New York Herald* in 1879 that the Utica crib was a barbarous torture device that was unsafe and dangerous for lunatics. He cited patients becoming more insane while contained in the crib and some dying in the device.

THE *AMERICAN JOURNAL OF INSANITY*

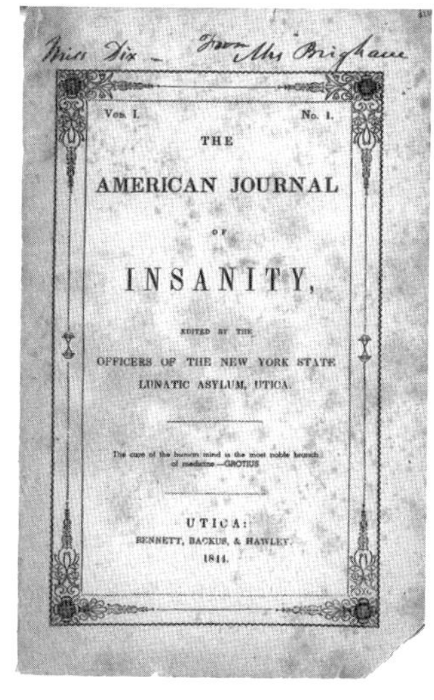
Miss Dix — From Mrs Brigham

Vol. I. No. 1.

THE AMERICAN JOURNAL OF INSANITY,

EDITED BY THE OFFICERS OF THE NEW YORK STATE LUNATIC ASYLUM, UTICA.

The care of the human mind is the most noble branch of medicine.—GROTIUS

UTICA: BENNETT, BACKUS, & HAWLEY. 1844.

The *American Journal of Insanity* was printed and published out of Old Main. *Oneida County History Center.*

The *Opal* is not the only publication that was written, edited and published at the Lunatic Asylum at Utica. The *American Journal of Insanity*, started in 1844 by Dr. Brigham, would attract the most brilliant minds and best writers in the field of mental illness. When Dr. Brigham passed away, the ownership was turned over to the asylum. This was the first journal published in the English language that was devoted to the study of mental illness. The journal dispelled fears and educated the public on all types of mental illness. The journal would continue to be published at the asylum until the 1890s, when it was purchased by the American Psychiatric Association. It was renamed the *American Journal of Psychiatry* in July 1921 but compiled, edited, written and published in the same print shop in Utica.

Patients of the Lunatic Asylum at Utica carefully read every issue of the journal and were compelled to write an editorial denouncing an article in the July 1859 issue. It was an article written by George Robinson, who favored a new system in the treatment of the mentally ill or "lunatics." He was proposing something different for the custody, discipline and managing of the insane. He had stated that places like the Lunatic Asylum at Utica were accumulating incurable patients and that a certain class of mentally ill should be considered "criminal" and classified as "violent passionate." The patients involved wrote in their opposition of this type of classification and asserted that Robinson wished a return of the mentally ill to almshouses, where there are no cures. The patients felt that Robinson wanted to create convict asylums.

The editors of the *Opal* considered this a regression of their treatment in the large state-built houses. They stated that those who commit simple assault are deemed mentally ill and not necessarily the same classification as those who have serious mental illness. They recalled that the old days of the treatment of mental illness largely involved hiding away people who were mentally ill in private homes, out of public view. They were victimized by people not qualified to provide proper care and in no way as qualified as the medical doctors providing treatment in large state-run facilities that had been erected to provide proper care. The interesting part of this debate is the response seems to go back and forth between "sheltered facilities" like Old Main, which had become the Utica Psychiatric Center, and the integrated settings and small community homes we have today.

Nathan D. Benedict, MD (1849–1854)

After the death of Dr. Brigham, first assistant physician Dr. George Cook served as interim superintendent until the arrival of Dr. Nathan Benedict, who came from Blockley Hospital in Philadelphia. Dr. Benedict had the stress of supervising the large asylum, and right after his start, in 1850, a suicide epidemic occurred. Suicide had always been a part of the asylum, but the numbers swelled in July 1850. He curtailed the number of suicides by putting more patients together and not in isolation. He had concluded that patients rarely killed themselves in the presence of other patients. Dr. Benedict continued the methodologies of Dr. Brigham on little or no restraints, and in 1852, he got rid of all the padded rooms and strong rooms. He was influenced by his new assistant physician, Dr. John Gray. This was considered a radical move at the time.

The asylum was only a decade old yet already in need of repairs and upgrades. Dr. Benedict had a thorough inspection conducted and deemed the asylum a fire hazard with poor ventilation due to the large wood-burning furnaces. The water supply was deemed inadequate. He was able to get appropriations of $28,000 from the legislature in order to convert the heating system to steam. The Lunatic Asylum at Utica would be the first facility of its kind in the United States to convert to the safer steam heat. The money also helped pay for improved ventilation by installing a mechanical fan blower, again the first institution to utilize such a device. The water supply increased and improved with supply by the Utica Water Works. Sanitary conditions were vastly improved with renovations of the bathing and toilet facilities. The greenhouse was enlarged, the farm had a new cow barn built and the lawns and trees were upgraded.

The asylum had a wonderful large chapel with a good organ that made a rich tone at Sunday services. The patients had among them many talented singers who filled out a wonderful church choir. The Reverend E.C. Goodrich, who had been the asylum chaplain since 1845, also experimented with fruits and vegetables, which led to vast improvement in the asylum's agriculture and horticulture. He earned the nickname "Utica's Burbank."

Dr. Benedict continued the occupational treatment that had all the shops working and making a profit. He started the successful *Opal*, which sold thousands of subscriptions and exchanges with hundreds of national periodicals that swelled the asylum with an assortment of reading material for the patients. Many amusements included patients partaking in games, music, dramatic performances and hosting visitors. The asylum became one of the largest tourist attractions in the United States in the 1850s, with over 2,700 visitors annually. There was great pride and public curiosity in Old Main.

Dr. Benedict allowed higher-functioning patients to travel out of the asylum for therapeutic visits to Utica fairs, Trenton Falls, outside church services and holiday celebrations. One stressor for which Dr. Benedict had no solution was the lack of separate quarters for the criminally insane, who were a danger to many of their fellow patients. Dr. Benedict appealed to the New York State legislature that a stand-alone facility for the criminally insane be built, since their mingling with other patients was putting some in danger and stressing the asylum staff. He suggested a facility that could host 250 would be of sufficient size. In 1854, the legislature repealed the act of 1846 that had committed the criminally insane to the asylum in Utica. It authorized this stand-alone facility in Auburn, New York, and had the criminally insane removed from the Lunatic Asylum at Utica.

Dr. Benedict found the job increasingly stressful and demanding, which affected his health, and he was forced to take a leave of absence. He went down south to more favorable weather and lifestyle conditions. He resigned in June 1854 and was succeeded by the brilliant and popular Dr. John Gray.

Annals and Recollections of Oneida County (1851)

In 1851, Pomroy Jones collected all kinds of statistics regarding Oneida County and compiled the data. Old Main is seated in Utica, New York, part of Oneida County, and Jones included some valuable information on the asylum. In 1850, there were 17,556 people living in Utica.

On March 30, 1836, an act was passed to create an asylum in New York State and the hiring of three commissioners to purchase land and oversee the construction. N. Dayton, C. McVean and R. Withers were the commissioners that reported to the legislature. The 130 acres was purchased in Utica, and then the legislature appointed Captain William Clarke of Utica, Francis E. Spinner of Herkimer and Elam Lynds to supervise the design, construction and erection of Old Main. Captain Clarke went and visited buildings that he thought might have the design he was looking for and used this to inspire his design for the asylum. The plan had originally a front of 550 foot in length, two side buildings and one back of the same distance. This would create a large courtyard of 13 acres in the middle.

The legislature approved funding to purchase furniture, fixtures, books, food, medicine, fuel and improving the grounds. One large improvement in 1843 was the construction of a drain that went down to the river that had provided water to the asylum. The water rate was 30 gallons per minute and moved by pumps up to a half mile. The water would be raised 95 feet up into a reservoir that was in the attic of the rear of the building. It was from here that water was moved throughout the asylum. Upon opening, the asylum admitted 276 patients in the first year. The amount of lunatics needing admission grew, so expansion was a must. The original additions were scrapped in 1844, and a wing off the main structure was constructed on each side 240 feet in length and 38 feet in width. The directors, legislators and New York citizens were overjoyed with the success and grandeur of Old Main.

Stats reported on February 25, 1851:

Patients remaining at end of last year:	226 males	223 females, for a total of 449
Admitted during the year:	185 males	82 females, for a total of 367
Patients discharged during the year:	94 males	77 females, for a total of 171

Much improved during the year:	4 males	4 females, for a total of 8
Improved:	26 males	23 females, for a total of 49
Unimproved:	51 males	57 females, for a total of 108
Died:	34 males	17 females, for a total of 51

Of the 171 who were discharged as cured, 124 had been insane less than one year, and 21 for one year, 9 for two years, 7 for three years, 2 each for years four and five, 1 for six years, and in 5 cases, the number of years insane had not been determined. Of the 51 deaths in the past year, 13 were from dysentery, 12 from chronic mania, 1 by suicide and 25 from 15 different diseases. The 816 patients came under different classifications, with 8 cases of fake insanity; 378 had been declared insane less than one year when admitted to the asylum, 277 insane from one to five years, 84 from six to ten years, 44 insane for eleven to twenty years, 21 declared insane, the remaining unknown.

The counties closest to the asylum had the largest number of patients admitted, with 287 from Oneida County, 102 from Madison County, 87 from Chenango, 94 from Jefferson, 79 from Herkimer, 55 from Erie, 46 from St. Lawrence, 33 from Dutchess and 21 from Delaware. The age of the insane admitted was 9 under the age of fifteen, 300 from the ages of fifteen to twenty, 953 from the ages twenty to thirty, 706 from the ages of thirty to forty, 451 from the ages of forty to fifty, 213 from the ages of fifty to sixty, 101 from the ages of sixty to seventy, 7 from the ages of seventy to eighty and 3 over the age of eighty. Occupation breakdown of those admitted to the asylum from 1843 to 1850 was as follows: of the men, 581 were farmers, 179 laborers, 71 merchants, 65 scholars, 47 joiners, 42 clerks, 16 clergymen, 24 lawyers, 20 physicians, 19 teachers, 36 shoemakers, 30 blacksmiths, 4 schoolboys; 1,167 women were engaged in housework, 52 schoolgirls, 35 tailor workers, 32 instructors, 28 mill workers, 21 mantua makers, 10 factory girls, 2 music teachers and 2 seamstresses. The rest were from a miscellaneous array of occupations.

The breakdown of the reasons for insanity of all patients admitted from 1843 to 1850 were listed as 448 cases of ill health, 205 cases of religious anxiety, 97 cases of lost property, 115 cases of puerperal, 110 cases of intemperance, 65 cases of disappointment in love (39 men and 26 women), 43 cases of Millerisma and 1 case each of the following: perfectionism, license question, Fourierism, preaching sixteen days and nights, mesmerism, visiting, smoking, anti-rentism, Rechabiteism, Mormonism and phrenology. There were 804 cases listed as unknown.

Suicide or suicidal tendencies were seen among the insane; with the 816 admitted, there were 66 identified as having made suicide attempts. The staff had to constantly watch them, and the sleeplessness and anxiety of these suicidal patients was noted. Dr. Benedict stated that the suicidal patients "form a burden which they alone know who bear it, increased by the necessity of carrying at all times, amid surrounding sadness, a cheerful countenance over a heavy heart." There was a suicide mania in July 1850. The mania was said to have been triggered by a single female patient, who, on July 12, 1850, became successful at self-destruction. She was listed as a favorite among the female ward, and her committing suicide sent many into a depression. The next day, staff overheard a plot by a group of the ladies to commit a suicide pact. An epidemic was brewing. One patient came close, as they had been discovered hanging themselves, were cut down and revived. One tried to cut her throat with a food utensil and another by ingesting a tincture of opium taken from an attendant. Another strangulation attempt occurred, and another patient tried to cut open a vein in her neck. For a two-week period, the suicide attempts among the women numbered fourteen, with staff stopping them from doing any more. Once August hit, the high rate of suicide attempts ended.

The *Opal*

A Monthly Periodical of the Lunatic Asylum

In the mid-nineteenth century, in the early days of the Lunatic Asylum at Utica, New York, the patients wrote and edited a series of publications called the *Opal*. These periodicals were written, printed and published right at the Old Main building from 1851 through 1859. Most of the authors remained anonymous, some with a single-word non de plume and others just a single initial or their first names. Some took on nonsensical names like Ichabod Artichoke and Jerusalem Ripestem. The periodical was sold to the public, and profits were used to purchase books for the asylum library, a piano and

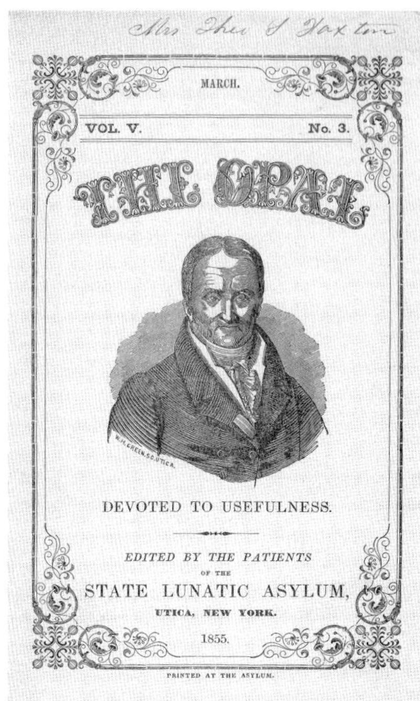

MARCH.

VOL. V. No. 3.

THE OPAL.

DEVOTED TO USEFULNESS.

EDITED BY THE PATIENTS OF THE STATE LUNATIC ASYLUM, UTICA, NEW YORK.

1855.

PRINTED AT THE ASYLUM.

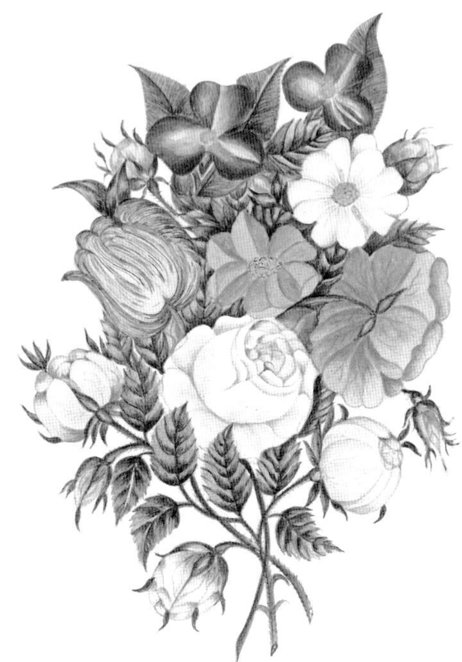

Left: *Opal* front cover featuring Pinel. Drawn by W.H. Green of Utica. *Oneida County History Center.*

Right: Flower drawing in the *Opal* by an asylum patient. *Oneida County History Center.*

an oil painting of Dr. Brigham. The publication proved very popular, with a peak of three thousand subscribers who paid one dollar per year for the monthly publication. Reading these volumes is an amazing experience and a treat I doubt few people have had the pleasure of partaking in. The *Opal* is full of poems, statements on modern events, observations on patient care, religion and politics. It's an eclectic collection and a perfect snapshot of the day-to-day lives of those who were confined by the walls of the Lunatic Asylum at Utica. Their hopes, dreams, frights and fears are all bound into a volume—people long since passed from this plane of existence. The one thing that cannot be tamed or restrained is the mind's eye wandering the universe and embracing the muse who runs words through the medium in the hand of the mentally ill. For their writings, their stories, their words, are to be admired. It was with awe that I carefully read the entire series of the *Opal*. The following is a collection of some of the incredible writings in this most valuable series:

Opal Disclaimer

The following blurb was written within the preface to the *Opal*, volume 9, 1859.

> *It is comforting ever in the storms to espy one ray of light—one intimation that all is soon to be well—that the hopes, the joys, the ambitions, the hatreds, the jealousies, the machinations of the world, are tinged with the immortal radiance of a divinity that sheds its glory around even reason,—the priceless gem that glitters in the Opal's diadem. It is the peculiar distinction and honor of the human race, and it is for it all the cares and anxieties, all the terrors of madness, all the misrepresentations of the ungracious, have here met and subdued unto the high and holy purpose of curing the insane. How noble is man!*

The disclaimer goes on to explain, excuse and ask forgiveness of readers and critics at the subject manner and literary weaknesses of the writing of the insane scribed, published and distributed to the masses. The authors asked for a kind reception to their heartfelt writings. The following are some of the best pieces I handpicked to replicate and comment on from the *Opal*, volumes 1 through 9, printed from 1851 to 1859.

It's important to note that those with high-functioning personalities were given the plumb occupations within the lunatic asylum. This included the writers, editor and printers of the *Opal*. The publications are filled with high praise for the staff and administrators, so one could easily read that the propaganda was strong to lean toward humane treatment, many cured patients bragging of wonderful experiences. In one letter by an ex-patient was printed the following: "I regard the Asylum as one of the most blessed Institutions that the 'Sarah' philanthropist has ever cause to existed. My recovery was due to extreme kindness and extreme care of which I was treated." In this day and age, it's easy to spot this sugar-coated public relations piece, but at the time it was important for the taxpayers to read that their investment in the asylum was yielding great human improved dividends. You can find little gems within the pages of the *Opal*, but never does the publication delve into the madness of the severely afflicted, locked in the isolation of the Utica crib, or any possible mistreatment. Most public tours rarely showed the bowels of the asylum, with most relegated to the rooms where the high-functioning patients resided. This doesn't diminish the fact that the *Opal* was written by the patients and revealed many items that have been plucked and placed within the pages of this book.

Editor's Table

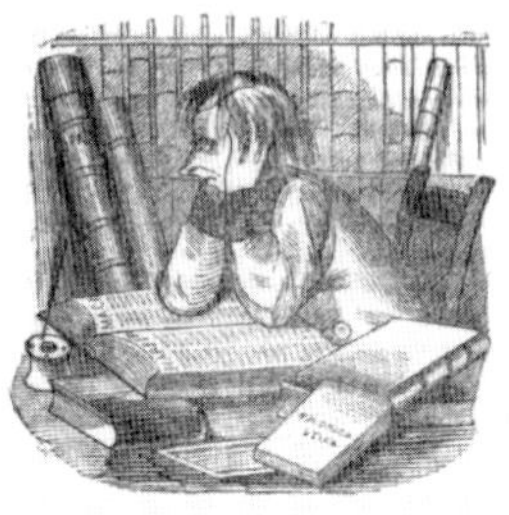

Opal editor, drawn by W.H. Green of Utica. *Oneida County History Center.*

This illustration was drawn by W.H. Green, Esq., and is in many of the *Opal* editions at the end of a section called "Editor's Table." The editors of the *Opal* were very pleased with the picture, yet Green stated he wished the face in his artwork had been a little handsomer. The editors felt the face was a wise one and it was better for it to look wise than handsome. An interesting side note: after the first few issues of the *Opal*, a man described as a "gentleman visitor" to the Asylum toured the print shop, the editor's room and then the library, where he stopped and remarked, "Ah, here is the *Opal* library." The visitor went along feeling the volumes, taking the books out of their nests, flipping the pages of the latest issue of the *Opal* and nodding in acceptance and said, "Well, really, that does not read so very much like as if it were written by an insane man after all." The editors took this as an insult to their craft.

Truthfulness with the Insane

In many parts of the *Opal*, the patients, who were the writers, editors and printers, offer opinion pieces. One on truthfulness leaps off the page, as you can feel the patients pleading with doctors to be truthful and not lie to patients about prognosis and possibility of recovery. The editors admit that people struggle to tell the truth all the time about everything but feel that physicians have an obligation to tell their patients the truth. They wrote, "An insane man is a man under the influence, commonly, of some bodily weakness or disease, and it is a very common effect of bodily sickness to produce, in a greater or less degree, mental derangement." The editors state that lying to patients about prognosis is the way of physicians and they had witnessed many times this tendency to deceive those with mental illness. They witnessed a doctor who would tell the truth to the family when not near the patient but would then stand next to the bedridden mental patient and tell them they would soon be completely healthy and recovered when there was no chance. The editors state that there are distinguished practitioners who do tell the truth but seem to lack honesty in regards to lunatics. They assert that placing delusion into the mind of the delusional is not a proper way to treat the insane. They do state that the insane who are told the truth and behave themselves are given certain privileges, including the freedom to walk; otherwise, they are restrained with devices like muffs and mittens that buckle down, solitary confinement and Utica cribs. Their theory is if doctors tell the truth, patients will accept it and then become more cooperative. There is no scientific data to back up any of these statements, simply the opinions of a group of patients who have the intelligence and skill to place pen to paper.

Pitying the Poets

Etta Floyd claims in her piece in the *Opal* a national pastime in giving pity to poets who are doomed to a life of misery, all due to dipping a quill into an inkwell and spilling thoughts on paper. She states that newspapers and magazines of the eighteenth century were filled with grotesque views and pathetic articles that focused on the affliction of the poet and not their wordsmith talents. She does claim truth in the long line of poets that had misery muses by stating:

> *Savage, it is true, was reduced to extreme indigence, which disheartening circumstance led him into a dissipated reckless course of life, that was at length terminated amid the horrors and the gloom of a prison. The youthful poet, Collins, from disappointed hopes became intemperate, and ere so long mentally diseased, that he was compelled to seek an abode in a lunatic asylum. Extravagance reduced Shenstone to penury, and what to a despairing lover was still worse, he was discouraged, and rendered irascible by an unreciprocated attachment. Akenside was crippled at an early age by the falling of a large hatchet upon his feet. Goldsmith was one upon whom fortune seldom smiled. He endured the extremes of poverty brought on by extravagance, and for a short time was immured within the walls of a prison. Chatterton, who distinguished himself, at an early age of eleven years, by his wonderful poetic talents, was reduced by adverse circumstances to poverty and degradation, and at last terminated his life by taking a potion of arsenic at the age of eighteen. Many, too, of our American poets fail not to receive a large share of pity.*

It's a compelling argument she makes about the intellectual weakness of the poet, as if it is in itself a mental condition to watch and write observations into verse.

Musings

In a piece written by Addison, we get a lecture on him being new to the lunatic asylum and his basic entry observations. He states that he has "membership" in the institution and that he is not a lunatic or insane. He critiques the *Opal* as possibly being of some usefulness to the lunatics. He felt that a mentally ill person was like a harp with a broken string and the institution should dedicate time and resources to repairing the mental instrument and not producing a periodical. Addison states that those who care for the mentally ill are of the highest moral order and have the richest quality of head and heart. He says they are doing the work of God. He adds the supervisor and managers have superior hearts and minds but also that the daily attendants, who were with the patients most of the time, are persons of worth and intelligence. Addison states that it's the obligation of the patients of the asylum to learn, and they should not seek perfection, as it is not attained, even by those not committed to a place of the insane.

Theaters

This piece was written by M.L. and lectures on the morality of the theater of the mid-nineteenth century. M.L. states that the gross and vulgar developments within the showcases were ruining the theater experience. M.L. claims evil minds were ruling theater operations and insidiously influencing and corrupting the viewing public. He speaks of the "moral Pecksniffs stealthily in the Lithean-like waters of contempt." He seems to be using a high moralistic view that in his psychosis was legitimate. He then goes on to state, "As it is now, theaters are but echoes of society development: they are mimic conventionalities; whereas, conventionality should be discarded; or be in subordination to ideality; - should be applied, not to reproduce human character as it is, but to convey an insinuation of what it ought to be." In his opinion, the theater is a stage for perfection and not human weaknesses.

M.L. goes on to chastise actors using voices different than natural ones. For instance, a male actor using the voice of an old woman is viewed as a "sing-song profanity." M.L. observes, "The actor may in his appropriate realm give free vent to the awe-inspiring workings of an emotional heart in tragedy, without intruding upon nonchalance of the statuesque bon ton; or allow his natural vivaciousness to unbend itself in sportiveness or spasmodic tomfooleries, without being at all conscious of having compromised his dignity." M.L. bases these observations on a trip he made with six other asylum patients to the Albany Museum to watch a play. Little did the actors of the time realize a critic was closely observing their performances.

The Ladies' Fair

The Lunatic Asylum at Utica housed adults, seniors and children of both sexes. On February 12 and 13, 1854, the asylum held a fair put on by the female patients and featured the hall fully decorated with evergreens and ferns. Remarks were made that the hall never looked better and all the tables had articles of usefulness and beauty that had been hand-crafted by the ladies of the asylum. The items were described as "transcendent loveliness." On one table was nothing but asylum literature and collections of poems, while the next table held flowers. A woman dressed in a fortune-teller costume gave positive outlooks. There was a table with a grab bag; patrons would pay a shilling, then reach into the bag and take out the prize, which was described as a baby doll. All ladies received the same prize. Another popular table was one that featured hand-made bonnets in every color and lace trim imaginable. There were many tables with needlepoint goods; all the while light music was played by the Asylum Band. The fair atmosphere was described as light and gay, and the asylum superintendent strolled around with a smile and a nod to the beauty. The ladies were of great spirit at the family and guest turnout at the fair. The attendants, of course, were in each corner of the hall, as if they felt the lunatics might not be satisfied with the barter. The ladies felt honored and privileged to have such benevolence in the face of the asylum. They praised the Lord God for the brisk attendance and generosity of the shoppers. A fine time was had by all in the great hall.

ROAD TRIP

Many letters to the *Opal* are from patients who had been released and wished to update friends remaining in the asylum. Most of these letters are unsigned, and the theory is the editors wished to keep names confidential, especially considering that the periodical was being sold to the public. One letter that was dated January 26, 1854, and sent from Albany, New York, was a lamentation from the author on people on the outside being more insane than the people locked up within the walls of the asylum in Utica. The man misses his friends and comforts yet has a companion whom he refers to as his "caregiver," so one can only assume this person is a guide to keep an eye on the mental particulars of the former patient. The letter writer goes on to describe riding in the "iron horse," or train, from Utica to Albany and how the last car was victim of a broken axle and the train had to be halted. All the passengers crammed into the remaining cars. There were no seats left, so men stood up and gave them to the women. The windows were frozen shut from the winter winds, and the heat supplied by stoves made the air light and thin. This caused many to gasp for air and threaten to put their canes through the windows. The writer goes on to describe the ladies as "superior" in their calmness and etiquette while the supposedly superior gender panicked, ranted and fumed in ill temper. The ex-patient found this most amusing and described the men as less rational and worse behaved than patients in the Lunatic Asylum in Utica. The writer departed in Albany and traveled with his companion to Massachusetts, where he raved about a large painting of Daniel Webster. But the highlight of the road trip was visiting and standing on Plymouth Rock. He found it quite amusing that a man went from being walled up in a lunatic asylum to plunking down on top of the landing of the Pilgrims.

UNCLE NICHOLAS'S DISCOURSES ABOUT FIRES AND FIREPLACES

This short piece written by patient Kathleen tells of her Uncle Nicholas and Aunt Mary lamenting about the decline of people having fireplaces to use as light, warmth and for cooking meals. All I can do is repeat it here word-for-word as it was written over 150 years ago. It's a fascinating documentation of modernization coming up against tradition:

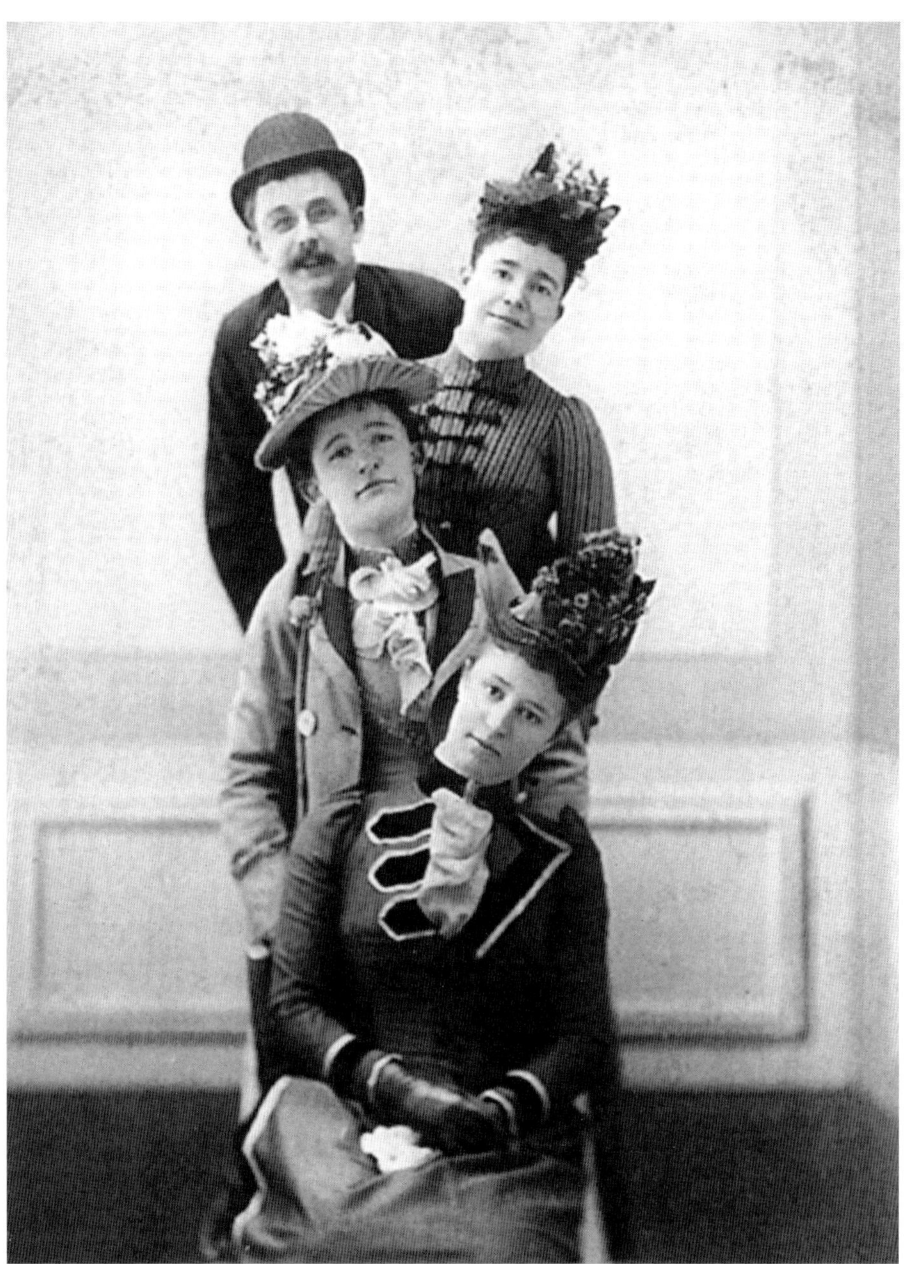

Visitors to the asylum. Old Main averaged over 2,700 visitors a year in the mid-nineteenth century, making it among the top tourist destinations in the United States.
New York State Archives.

> *I pity people who have only stoves to work and sit by; it gives me a sad feeling to see a fine fire-place shut up and a black stove in its place, and it gives me a headache as well as a heartache. I don't pity some of them, because they might know better, and it makes me indignant, to see me who call themselves sensible, pull down good old-fashioned chimneys, with ample fire-places, and put in health-destroying stoves and furnaces; miserable, grim, unsmiling, unsociable stoves, or, instead of that, a set of poisonous holes in their floors, called registers.*

Kathleen goes on to discuss her visiting a prominent physician friend and the horror she encountered in walking into the mansion at the acrid and villainous breath being spewed forth by the good doctor's new furnace. She found the doctor's wife and daughters warming their feet on the metal grid on the floor they called the "register." Kathleen fled the home in fear and vowed not to return.

For some of these claims, there can be no verification, as some could be 100 percent true and others could be the ramblings of a madman or madwoman, but it does not dull the effect nor change the outcome of their afflictions. One does, upon reading these writings in the *Opal*, get the sense that the patients believed in what they were writing. The record gives a full portrait of people, who, although confined for their afflictions, led full lives filled with interesting experiences. In the "Editor's Table" of volume 9, they write of the patients having their own musical group called the "Lunatic Band." The Lunatic Band practiced one song at a time and would play that single song for half a day, over and over until they could play it to perfection. A group of theater performers put on shows for the viewing public right inside the walls of the asylum at Utica. They also wrote of a young lady from the "Women's Wing" of the asylum who had been in four previous asylums but found Utica, in 1859, to be by far the best in terms of life and surroundings, especially the lavish greenhouse that city visitors praised regarding its beauty, the splendor of the plants and the glorious scents of the flowers.

Asbestos

In the *Opal*, the name Asbestos appears regularly as the non de plum of a prolific writer and possible historian. They wrote of the sixteenth anniversary, a Sunday, from the opening in 1843; due to religious services and observation of the Sabbath, the patients were able to conduct a celebration on the Monday next. The asylum supervisor made a speech, and the Asylum Band played many songs and marches to great fanfare. It's after this pomp and circumstance that Asbestos stood up in front of the gathering of patients, staff, administration and visitors to raise praise and blessings for the charitable state and benefactors who gave greatly in order for the patients to gather together and enhance their lives. Asbestos praised the architecture of Old Main, the wisdom and virtue within the walls. "Insane lunatic hearts swell with love and gratitude," said Asbestos, to loud applause. Asbestos finished the address by waving a hand at the assembled group and stated, "These poor renovated insane are our jewels!" It's interesting that within the *Opal*, names of the doctors are rendered as "Dr. M-----e," or any lawyers as "Esq. B-----e." It's not mentioned if this non-naming was to keep the reading public from knowing the names of the staff or if it was a mandate by the administration.

Mr. and Mrs. Santa Claus and Baby Orville

In volume 4 of the *Opal*, which came out in 1854, is a letter written by a patient describing a wonderful Christmas party that had a gathering of staff, administration and the patients in a room where music was played and food and drink distributed. The occasion brought about gay and happy times, laughing, singing and doing what the patients described as "tripping the light fantastic." A bell rang that brought about silence. After a dramatic pause, Mr. and Mrs. Santa Claus came walking into the room, with Mrs. Claus carrying in her arms a baby that the patients assumed was the child of the Christmas couple. Mrs. Claus handed the baby off to patients, who took turns dancing with the baby in their arms. Mrs. Claus announced the baby's name was Orville. Mr. and Mrs. Claus danced to the joyous music while the patients took turns kissing baby Orville. The patients described Orville as sweet, pretty and amusing. Little Orville brought great joy to the patients of the lunatic asylum, as babies and children were rarely seen, let alone held by the patients, especially those who had been confined for many years.

A Chapter from Real Life

The only attribution to the author is "written by an ex-patient." This letter written to the *Opal* was one of heartbreak and describes a human being who had been tormented with mental illness, was placed in the Lunatic Asylum at Utica, recovered and went on to live their life outside the confines. The patient writes in their letter that it had been two years since they had been released from the asylum. They describe the horror they lived. When the mental illness started, the patient was hearing voices and sought solace in a local graveyard, where they describe the voices of the dead speaking to them. They state they suffered from mental blindness and that they had prayed to God to help them. The patient had a fear of eating for fear of choking, so they were eating three meals every two weeks. The patient was having night terrors and envisioned themselves as evil and not worthy of God. The parents placed the mentally ill child in the Lunatic Asylum in Utica, where the patient feared death among gawking strangers. The patient came to loathe their parents' overly religious lectures and felt at peace with and loved Dr. Brigham, whom the patient felt was a gentle soul, a smiling angel who ran the facility yet showed great compassion for the patients under his care.

The writer felt better at the asylum but still felt tortured by what they called the soul of a woman. The patient had felt they deserved to be punished, so they held their fingers under scalding hot water until all the tips of their fingers had the skin peeling off. They felt they were regressing into a fiend and stopped attending all religious services. Their evil body should not be crossing the threshold of a holy place. They were given to writing along with the *Opal* staff and started to feel better and even partook in a Thanksgiving meal, yet afterward guilt flooded them and they openly wept, to the confused looks of colleagues and staff. It was that night that the patient describes being locked in his room, in bed, experiencing darkness, and just when the blackness enveloped them, they were visited by a bright light that was an epiphany. They were good after all. They sensed the love and gratitude of what could only be described as a guardian angel that had come down and embraced them. The patient couldn't describe what had happened as the love changed them. Within months, they had been released, never to return. Their final words to his friends, still in the asylum, were, "I only know that whereas I was blind…I now can see."

Asylum Entertainers

On February 19, 1857, the patients put on an entertainment spectacle that also included some of the attendants. The Asylum Band accompanied the performance with music. One of the patients painted the stage backdrop that was described as a wooded scene featuring wildlife, trees and water. There was an additional backdrop that featured a ship struggling in the rough waters of the open sea. The editors of the *Opal* drew the analysis that the ship at sea represented their own lives in conflict with the norm. The Asylum Band performed the overture from the opera *Anna Bolena*. The *Floral Tableau* was performed by six women adorned in pure white gowns. After a series of musical performances, a group of several staff and patients performed *The Oddity*, which was billed as a parlor comedy and lasted forty minutes. This was followed by an Irish comedy and a Yankee performance called *Old Ladies Visit* that was met with roars of laughter. It seems the patients and staff were mocking the behavior and reactions of elderly women who visited the lunatic asylum. The conclusion was a ballet performance that roused the house and was a tribute to Pocahontas. The performances were met with loud applause. Among the attendees were the board of directors, who were described as stodgy gentlemen yet had cracked smiles on their stoic faces. It was an overwhelming success and a glimpse that among the patients were those who possessed a premium in musical, comedy, singing, writing and painting talent on par with that of any sane troupe.

About a Patient

This essay was written by a patient at the Lunatic Asylum who never identified himself. He only says it was written "By Himself." He put pen to paper in February 1857 and says that one year prior he had been with his parents on the family farm on Long Island and in excellent mind and body. He says his weight was a healthy 150 pounds and he was nineteen years old. He had been cheerful and content with his work on the farm, which had consisted mostly of chopping wood during the winter and taking part in a debating society that challenged his mind. It was at this point that he had become interested in religious meetings at his local church. He attended them every night, walking back and forth in freezing cold weather. He claims the small, hot room was too crowded with people, all talking loudly, which caused him agitation.

After ten days of this, he claims he suddenly was unable to sleep and paced his room all night long. He went four days without sleep and was chopping wood when he got lightheaded and dizzy. Afterward, he could not help himself and began talking nonstop and rapidly. He began to get paranoid and became starved from not eating. The constant talking continued until he became bedridden. Slowly, his strength came back, first from fluids, then from solid food. Then his visions began: the sun shining at the foot of his bed with clouds floating by. When he was finally able to descend the homestead stairs, he'd stare at flowers and see hundreds of golden crosses and Bibles. He started to sit in the window all day and watch the children and animals playing in the field next to his house. Finally, someone mentioned the Lunatic Asylum in Utica. His aunt had been there, and he recalled her speaking of the freaks and fancies that had been within. His brother took him to a steamboat that brought him upriver to the asylum. He ended up bedridden at the asylum and tried to ignore the voices and cries that were echoing down the hall. The sweet music of the Asylum Band would perk him up. He mentions the sweet doctor who spoke at his bedside and told him he'd recover. He eventually recovered enough that he was put to work on the asylum farm and much enjoyed tending to it and building the fences that penned in animals. He finally spoke after several months of silence and started playing games of checkers with his fellow patients. In the last line of his essay, the patient states that he is feeling well enough that he had hoped they would release him and let him go home. We can only hope he got his wish to be released and taken back home.

Daily Life at the Asylum

An article was written by a person listed only as H. Their mundane daily life is written about and mentions that people are admitted into their "hotel" daily and come from different places and arrive in different manners. They state that the asylum hotel has no superior in the United States and the patients called the arrivals "fashionables," although others would refer to this mental class as "unfortunates." It's stated that a patient's hotel bill had to be paid in full and signed by the superintendent before they could check out. Both sexes are at the asylum but live on what is referred to as "Shaker

Principals [*sic*].” This means everything is strictly scheduled and regulated. The bell rings at five o’clock in the morning to alert all to rise from their beds. This, of course, did not apply to those patients sick in their beds or confined to Utica cribs. There is always food to eat, even if the patients lack money. The writer of this daily life list states that bedtime was strictly at 8:30 p.m. and all hotel guests were locked in their rooms—only to keep them from leaving without paying their bill. On Sundays, there are church services in the chapel, which is the only time the male and female patients are together. Monotony is usually deflected by game playing, although there was a rule of no card playing. Music is a great entertainment, with all sorts of musical acts performing for the patients, including the Christys, the Campbells, the Euphonians, young Paul Julien and more. Sometimes the Asylum Band played or individual resident musicians would take the stage. Although life in the Lunatic Asylum at Utica is portrayed as dull, the writer does use the sympathy of the reader to solicit them paying for a subscription to the *Opal*. Only, of course, so the readership would know of the amenities at the hotel.

Lunatic Marriage Ad

The June 1856 edition of the *Opal* featured an ad placed by an actual patient secured within the asylum walls. She had placed an ad wanting to get married. The ad is littered with misspellings, but the editors kept the letter word for word. Here is exactly how it appeared more than 150 years ago:

> *To Eny Body and Evry Body*
> *Utica, March the 21, 1856*
>
> *This is to certify that I am a woman in my 30 fifth year I want to get married I will Have eny Man that will have me matters not whether he has wif or not I have auburn hair black eyes Blunt nose thick Lips Look rather young if I had not lost my teeth look as well as eny body that dont look eny better than I do my hight is five fete three Inches weight generly one Hundred 24 pounds can scold things well if things dont go right Residence Utica Asylum (signed)*
>
> *N.B. Please put this up in some publick place or coppy it off I would like it put in the papers in Print if you think I know what I want.*

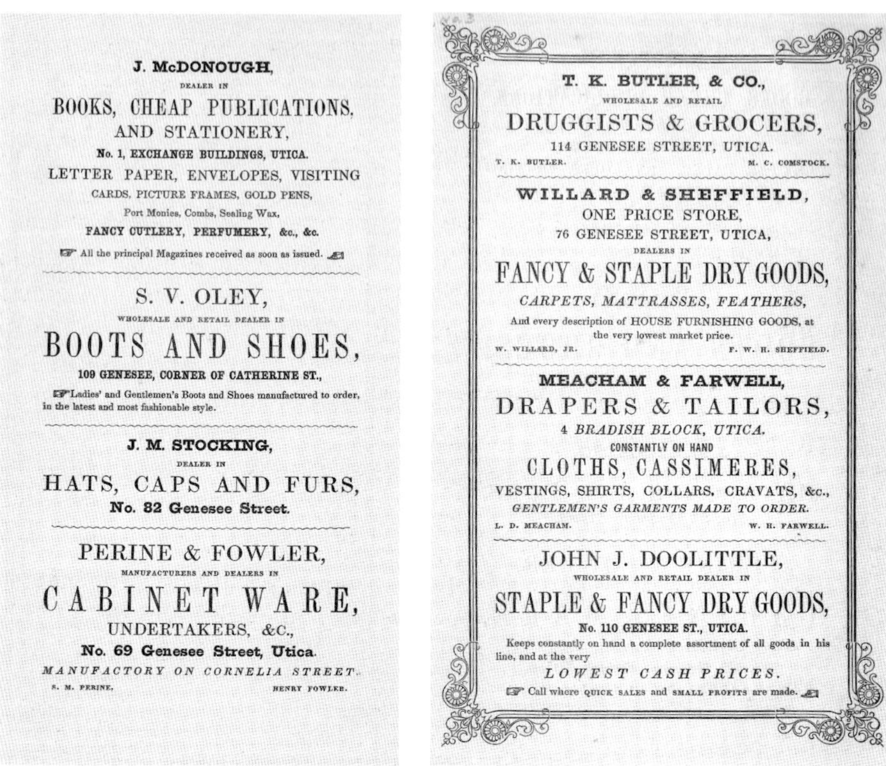

Left: The *Opal* received paid advertisements from Utica merchants. *Oneida County History Center*.

Right: *Opal* ads. The monthly peaked at over three thousand paid subscribers. *Oneida County History Center*.

Bon Mots

Here are some vignettes of daily life and observations taken from the *Opal*, volumes 1 through 9:

The Zavistowiski Troupe of a dozen Polish Infantry youth visited the asylum and performed for the patients by dancing on a small stage. They showed great cheerfulness and cheer, for the patients especially became enamored with the littlest performer, an energetic five-year-old girl named Alice. The children were allowed to run up and down the halls of the asylum to the great joy of the patients. The performers also stopped to see the Ladies Fair showcase and came away with mementos of their visit.

An anonymous lady in the women's wing observed with great joy out her window the sight of winter sleighs gliding through the powdery winter snow along the Whitesboro Road. She greatly enjoyed listening to the ringing bells and clapping hooves on the packed snow and witnessing the huffs of breath snorted via the nostrils of the bounding horses.

A group of people who were unable to speak visited the asylum in January 22, 1856, and was described in the *Opal* as "Visit of the Mutes." The visitors were being escorted by a Mr. Skinner, who was traveling with the group to Minnesota, where they had planned on establishing a deaf and dumb asylum. It was a small group that included the leader, his wife, Mrs. Skinner, a Mr. Grow, a deaf-mute man and his wife. They had in their micro-flock one little girl and three little boys who did not speak. Mrs. Skinner led the group by reciting the Lord's Prayer while the visitors interpreted with their hands and faces. The children then did a series of pantomimic imitations of humans, animals and birds, among other things. They mesmerized the asylum patients and drew gasps of admiration and applause of appreciation. The *Opal* mentions the visitors were "the human face divine" and "an eloquence of nature." The talents on display left an impression on the patients as they marveled at the captivating gifts.

The ladies of the asylum, being in their own private wing and separated from the men except for church services or a formal event, had to stave off cabin fever and boredom by resorting to children's games. The most amusing to them was playing "Puss in the Corner." Though it was a game said to be for the young, the ladies of the first hall found it not only fun but also the most joyful period in their time in the asylum.

The asylum offered many religious avenues for patients, including church services at the on-site chapel and plenty of religious writing in the *Opal*. Some patients were allowed to leave the asylum to go to local churches for their religious services, but some had only the in-house service. A chaplain referred to as Mr. Sanford was claimed to have been the first preacher in the country to preach to mentally ill patients with services geared toward them. The patients referred to him as a valuable and worthwhile person with wonderful sermons. In one autumn address, he said that citizens and patients were like the leaves on a tree in the fall: they started out green and fresh and then made a rapid transition to fall foliage, die, then flitter to the ground. He ended his sermon with the assertion, "We all do fade as the leaf." The patients referred to Mr. Sanford as a "fine old man."

The asylum farm and garden was tended by the patients with love and care and had all sorts of fruits, vegetables and flowers. The Oneida County

Fair of 1851 featured many flowers, fruits and vegetables from farmers all over the county and included a cornucopia of offerings from the asylum. The cabbage and celery from the asylum garden were highly praised and won the "premium" award from the judges.

Editors and writers of the *Opal* came across a young male patient of the asylum who was sitting in a corner reading a book that had been donated—one of six hundred volumes in the library. They asked what the lad was reading, and it was a book of poetry. The young boy looked up, smiled and said, "This is a wonderful book. It has a picture in it. The poems are not as good as the *Opal* but I like it anyway."

Interested patients were taken on a road trip to the Mechanic's Fair in Utica to see one thousand different manufactured devices on display in the Mechanics Hall. They were thrilled to see these manufactured items of all variety and skill, along with the entertainment being delivered by the Utica Brass Band. The patients marveled at all the crafts, paintings, machines and many items handcrafted by the residents of Oneida County.

Daniel Webster, the famous attorney, is mentioned with great fondness within the pages of the *Opal*. And there was great joy when Professor Noyes, who had been Webster's classmate, arrived at the Lunatic Asylum at Utica with a gift: a lightning rod. The patients gathered around to shake hands with Professor Noyes or touch the lightning rod with admiration before it was placed on top of Old Main.

There was a theft at the asylum that was referred to as "Strayed or Stolen": the missing item was a neat little metallic box with a drawer, a cover and the Skenondogh seal on the bottom. It states that the box had contained several coins of different dates, including a dime that was from 1839; that the coin had been a gift from a very distinguished person. Also inside were bank notes, including one valued at forty dollars, which was a lot of money in those days. There was another bank note valued at eighty dollars, a half-dime, a sixpence dated 1789 along with California gold and rubies. The loser of this box may well be exaggerating the value and items inside, but they did mention that they had contacted Sheriff Bell, the undersheriff of Fairfield County, and Honorable Esquire Gillmore, who lived "upstairs." The box's owner claimed that the finder of the box would be rewarded and paid "accordingly."

An odd letter came into the *Opal* from Araminta C. Stubbs. The editors printed it, but the missive was nothing but a lamentation on a visit that had been a disappointment. Stubbs said that she and her friends decided to take a sleigh ride into Utica to see the lunatic asylum and arrived after dark. The guard at the front door refused admittance. She and her merry party were offended and stated they didn't come to just stand underneath the large stone pillars but to have free admission and a tour of the place. The guard excused himself, and another man, who was stated as handsome, came and allowed them to walk the halls but asked them to please be respectful. Stubbs complained in her letter that the patients were strolling around acting normal and that was not what they were there to see. Plus, she was upset that the asylum was clean and begged her good-looking guide to show them something. He cordially walked them to their sleigh, tipped his hat and bid them goodbye. She stated in her letter that she was very upset and would never come back and intended to tell all her friends to never visit unless they were allowed to see something of a lunatic. In her postscript she asked the name of the handsome guide and wondered if he were a patient.

Funds used to publish and print the *Opal* were stolen, and the latest volume requested their return. Back in 1859, paper money was issued by individual banks. The notes in question were described as "two very good looking bills, one $10 bill and one $1 bill, not filled up and issued by the Red Hook Building Company."

A listing in the *Opal* offered a reward of one dollar for the return of the collar of the asylum dog, Snuffy. The collar had a padlock on it with an inscription, "I am the State's dog; whose dog are you?" The patients set the reward as one dollar. They said that the original amount was two dollars, but since the pistol that killed Hamilton cost one dollar they could not have the reward higher, although they were offering a reward of forty-nine dollars for the capture of the highway robber. The patients stated in the ad that the dog "has done the state, not some, but much service, and so highly do we patients deplore this loss, and resent the indignity and outrage offered to the person of Snuffy that we offer this one dollar reward." They described Snuffy as the "chattel appurtenant" of the institution. The friendly pup would walk among the eaters in the dining hall wagging his tail and receiving scraps from the patients. He was described as mischievous and a universal favorite in the asylum.

Many bands came to the Asylum to entertain the patients, and only those who were sane enough or well behaved could attend in the hall. On one occasion in 1852, there was a minstrel band that was most impressive, especially the banjo player. The *Opal* noted the fact the band was called the Nightingales and had prepared themselves as "darkies," which means they were performing in blackface. Minstrel shows were very popular in the United States. They were described as "accomplished artists who tripped the light fantastic while personifiers of the dark race." Another minstrel group came right after, the Ethiopian Minstrels of Mr. Fellows, the blackface performers praised as tender, sincere and most musical. It was not unusual at the time for traveling musicians to partake in such racial theatrics, yet the highest praise was for a band made of people who were blind. The visually impaired vocalists were remarkable in their singing skills and performed with great zeal inside the walls of the lunatic asylum. They were praised for their admirable skill despite their disabilities and were from a school for the blind, which was highly praised as something unique in this world.

The editors wrote about the number of Black people in the slave states and fully supported freedom and expansion of rights to those who were oppressed under the umbrella of slavery. The patients locked up, most against their own wishes for freedom, had great sympathy for those held against their will. The editors felt that many in the country were interested in abolition and the formerly enslaved being allowed to take part of the colonization.

The segregation of men and women was mentioned, but integration of the two sexes occurred during soirees, the Sabbath, exhibitions or other appointed events by the administration and then only those who were sane enough to be cordial and well mannered. Otherwise, most everything was in separate wings.

The cupola was a glorious spot that was shown to many visitors, who would look out from the highest point of the asylum and view Utica and the surrounding area in all their glory. A young woman patient by the name of Miss Spencer had gained access, as patients were not allowed up there. She escaped her keepers and bolted up to the apex of the asylum and threw herself from the top, committing suicide. A student visiting the asylum from Hamilton College wrote an essay on the event that included the line "swift as the lightning of heaven she darted into eternity."

A college diploma delivered to a patient at the asylum was described in the *Opal* as a "veiled mystery." Even though it had been deemed an "honorary diploma," it came from Old Yale and went to what was listed as a "senior resident" of the asylum. It conferred this man the honorary degree of Doctor of Medicine. There was great discussion on how the diploma had been delivered: submarine, telegraph, Underground Railroad or by some metamorphosis without hands. They carefully examined the diploma and deemed it beautiful and genuine. The mystery was never solved but caused quite the stir among the patients, staff and faculty.

Medical quackery is nothing new even in our modern age, but in the mid-nineteenth century, many snake-oil salesmen rode the trails and tramps pitched their wares for cures for everything from consumption to pox. Well, it was talked about among the patients at the asylum the quack treatments that had been tried and applied, and one story that stood out was of a peddler trying to offer cures to parents for their insane children. It was a concoction of wild cherry, snakeroot and mullein that reportedly tasted pleasant, and as long as the parent forced the child to drink it on a regular basis, the child's mental illness would be cured. As long as children kept drinking the elixir they would stay cured. The parents would spend all they had to make their children sane, and one had ended up at the Lunatic Asylum at Utica, where the parents were heard telling the tale of the quack. The snake-oil salesman quipped to the parents of the mentally ill child, "Let all the world quit all Patent Medicines, and take mine."

Editors of the *Opal* took great offense at being called "crazy head" by a member of Congress and compared the inmates in the Lunatic Asylum at Utica to the behavior of members of Congress. The editors stated that at least the asylum cures people and sends them home with newfound sanity and asked if the Congress lunatics could brag of the same.

An article titled "Grand Preliminary Caucus" recorded a political meeting hosted by the patients where they invited a veteran of two U.S. wars, but the specific engagements are not mentioned. This grizzled veteran appeared in the great hall at the asylum and spoke to the assembled patients about "rotten ruins of the old party." The patients came from the meeting with a platform in which they asked for three simple items: 1) Bring back the simple principles put forth in the Constitution as administered by George Washington, 2) end slavery by peaceful means but by force if necessary and 3) classify and distinguish the efforts of the insane. The group gave themselves the name the Sane Party.

A group of men were assembled watching two men in a battle of checkers when a group of visiting ladies stopped and remarked to the asylum administrator, "Do you think they understand the moves?" This query resulted in a hearty group laugh by the crowd of male spectators.

"Our Horses!" is an article that mentions the two horses that belonged to the asylum and were used to transport people and haul goods. Charlie and Jerry were called lovely cream-colored brothers with sleek coats, dark brown manes and tails and "flashing eyes." The two horses had been driven side by side since colthood. Charlie was known as the fleet one and Jerry as the more powerful. The pair easily hauled 1,500-pound loads to and from the train depot. Their breed is mentioned as a mix of Devonshire, Durham and Yankee. The longtime driver of the pair affirmed the feelings of the asylum patients: Charlie and Jerry were the best horses in the land.

The asylum chapel was visited by a traveling group of African Americans the editors of the *Opal* referred to as "Ethiopians" who played musical instruments. The gathered patients were especially captivated by the banjo playing of one of the group. Afterward, the superintendant asked a group of patients how they enjoyed the entertainment, and one responded, "The pulpit looked very well, very well indeed."

The gift of a billiards table by Michael Phelan was met with great appreciation and fanfare, as the asylum convalescents' happiness would be greatly enhanced. They mention Washington Irving having a fondness for the game and were also appreciative of a book titled *A Manual on the Game of Billiards* written by Phelan. The donor, in addition to the billiards table and the book, gave a sum of $400 for the proper care of the patients, which was a grand sum back in 1859. The patients became so skilled at pocket billiards that a professional visited and lost a match when one patient made fifty-one straight shots. It was not long after this that a pamphlet titled *On the Evils of Gaming*, by Reverend E.H. Chapin, appeared.

An unnamed patient lamented the freedom of the robin bounding around the green grass with its red breast and its trill. The bird had the freedom to move about and enjoy the outside; the patients had recently been denied the freedom to walk the grounds of the asylum untethered.

In the spring of 1854, Benjamin Plant of New Hartford, New York, presented a gift to the asylum in the form of two deer. The asylum already had one doe with a newly born fawn, and the patients were overwhelmed and overjoyed at the graceful gift and praised Plant.

A group of patients was engaged in a late-night game of "Hurly Burley," in which the rules of the game seem to be similar to truth or dare. It was during this game that an Irish guard, walking the squid ink nighttime asylum halls with his lit candlestick, came upon several patients. It was described as a shocking sight by the Irish-born night watchman, whose jaw dropped before he lit into what the patients figured was foul ranting, yet none understood. The Irishman ripped off a language streak in his native Irish tongue. Needless to say, the game ceased, and the patients were escorted back to their beds. with the night watchman wondering how the patients had unlocked their rooms.

Among the farming and other outside activities, the patients were enthralled with the buzz and hum coming from the large beekeeping area.

In addition, it was noted that there were fifteen different tree species on the Utica grounds, yet the most excitement was saved for the abundant crop of horseradish. The asylum grounds were tended by the patients with gentle care and great love.

A patient wandering the grounds up past the farm, in the area where Utica College now sits, discovered mineral spring waters, which was named "Asylum Spa." The waters were described as sparkling, transparent and holding minerals of iron and sulphur (sulphurous gas). The staff surmised that there were other healing minerals present within the water. The patients lucky enough to have freedom to wander the grounds drank from the Asylum Spa and described the water as light and pleasant to the taste. It was described as being on the edge of the property in a northwestern direction, next to a ravine. The patients wondered if the Asylum Spa would become a place of healing for residents of Utica.

Calico ruffles, the hottest fashion of 1859, were described as "utterly distasteful" by the editors of the *Opal.* They called this collar unbecoming, preposterous, lacking taste and common sense. "It's all the fashion" said visitors to the lunatic asylum, but the editors felt the "good old way" of wearing a neat white collar would not detract from a lady's beauty. "Hoops! Hoops! Hoops!" is the headline of one article in which the editor of the *Opal* stated the newest women's fashion is an amusing scene, but worthy ladies would be best to stay with traditional garb. Then again, the hoop-wearing ladies were causing quite the spectacle and amusement among the patients of the asylum, especially the men, who would call out to "de-hoop" the ladies wearing the daring fashion. In an 1854 piece, the new teardrop-shaped earrings were criticized as well as ladies wearing headdresses that came halfway down the forehead. This was called a "trifling addition to a dress." The new rage of wooden shoes that were clunky but helped shape ladies' feet were not highly thought of, even though they had liners of pink or blue lush. The one praise was the new creation of sewing a blue or cherry-colored ribbon to the end of handkerchiefs in order to make them easier deployed.

The patients of the lunatic asylum were honored to be able to go on the road to New Hartford, New York, to watch and partake in the celebration of the Battle of Bunker Hill. There were one thousand residents and visitors to the celebration, where silence fell while the preacher said a prayer for the fallen and the good graces of the aftermath of the battle. It was a celebration of a battle for freedom. The group prayed for the souls of those who sacrificed their blood on the battlefield. The asylum visitors were most thankful to be able to be away from their confinement and to witness a ceremony that celebrated Washington and his brave horde.

An unnamed patient at the lunatic asylum wrote that he had "special illusions" in his insanity. He beheld a four-legged turkey and observed kitten-butterflies in the air around the grounds, yet the writer's lament was not being home in Ratville by the side of Crooked Lake writing to stricken lunatics.

Professor B. Yates's Ballet and Pantomime Troup visited the lunatic asylum on May 28, 1856, and put on a show that the patients loved. The dancers performed on the stage to a packed room and commented they had never performed in such a place for such a crowd. The dancers performed and then offered their sympathies to the afflicted. The performances of the ballet dancers and the pantomimes were described as elegant, beautiful and entertaining. The patients thanked them for their performance and kindness and wished them the best of luck and success on the rest of their tour.

Thanksgiving was a special occasion at the asylum, with an abundance of turkeys, geese, pies and tarts served to the patients followed by Professor Shaw playing favorite tunes on the piano. The Asylum Band soon took to their instruments, prompting many patients to get up and dance and causing quite a stir among the stern Yankee patients.

Ladies at the asylum had great fondness for the tomatoes grown in the patient garden and called them "love-apples." One particular patient of the asylum wore an apron with deep pockets and would be seen strolling the grounds with her pockets laden with the freshly picked tomatoes—so much so that they were observed falling out and rolling across the floor. Then the apron lady would carry the largest of the crop in her hand and stop her stroll to take a small bite of the delicious love-apple, declaring it the most delicious thing ever tasted.

The *Opal* was a hit publication, with subscribers coming in from every state of the union and some writing letters to the editors amazed that a well-written paper could come from a group with mental disabilities. The editors assured their subscribers that people from the asylum could indeed write literate content and solicited donations or bartered; all those who wished to have an exchange would receive a copy of the *Opal*. The paper had over one thousand subscribers. The editors did compare their plight to Napoleon and wondered what the sane people in the outside world would think if they had a revolution inside the thick walls and locked gates of the asylum. They claimed that someday in the future this would happen and those with "non-cracked brains" shall rue the day.

The Asylum Band responded to a critique by the institutionalized ladies that they had not played for the women for quite some time. They wondered if it was the heat of the summer or their shyness of performing in front of female eyes. Band members responded to this query by humbly apologizing, as in the summer of 1859, their band lost a few key members. Some had been released from the asylum, and new members were practicing. They did not want to perform until they were prepared to do so and asked by the patients to play their violins and guitars.

The asylum's Dramatic Corps performed entertaining skits and musicals for the administration, staff and patients. One particular evening, they were enthralled by a performance of the burlesque tragic opera *Bombastes Furioso*, which was described as being delivered in the "Burton style." The musical arrangements were played by the Asylum Band. The opera was performed to great amusement, and laughter rang through the hall.

There was a touching tribute to a female patient who passed away in 1856 whose name was Kathleen. She died in her bed in the night. The writer of the tribute mentioned that the asylum was quiet for days and there had been hushed voices all around. Kathleen must have been a beloved person, for the writers refer to her as "the fairest flower that hath gone onto heaven where she could bloom for eternity." They wished her well in her peaceful release and stated she was now free and happy in heaven.

There was a wedding ceremony at the asylum in August 1856. Dr. Chatfield and his wife were visiting the asylum from Nashville, Davidson County, Tennessee, where the doctor was the superintendent of the Tennessee Asylum for the Insane. They were traveling home after attending a superintendant conference. They had visited the Lunatic Asylum at Utica in the past, and all had been impressed with the family, including their beautiful daughter. So much fondness was there that the Chatfields held their daughter's wedding at the asylum. Their eldest daughter married a man described only as Mr. Hathaway. The ceremony was performed by the Reverend Mr. Leeds, rector of Grace. The asylum friends and patients attended the ceremony, and a poem was read, "Marriage, rightly understood, Gives to the tender and the good. A paradise below."

A group of patients on the grounds of the asylum during a warm summer evening was treated to something that caused the patients to laugh. They said that "the change induced in our cerebral tissues, was an excitation of the special organ of mirthfulness, which was instantly reflected into that complication of nerve-and-muscle machinery necessary to the phenomenon of a hearty laugh." The patients mentioned that the laughter went a long way to ease their homesickness. The tale is as follows. The group stood at the edge of the property by Whitesboro Road and observed a tidy milch cow twelve rods in front of a loitering, lagging young boy. The cow had stopped and was eating grass on the side of the road, when a boy and a girl had scrambled underneath the animal. They were holding their cupped hands under the udder and were milking handfuls that they quickly scooped up to their mouths. Upon observing the thieves, the owner stood upright and ran fast to the cow, yelling out, "Hey! Hey there! What'r' y'r bout? Stop that—stop milking that cow!" The two urchins came from underneath with palms to mouths and didn't speak until they were done slurping, took their hands away from their mouths, smiled and said, "Soak your head, Benny!"

"The Life of Vegetation"

The *Opal* was open to submissions from former patients of the Lunatic Asylum at Utica, and one of note is "The Life of Vegetation," written by Ichabod Artichoke. In this essay, he stated that he was a bona fide vegetable and had gained consciousness only a few years prior. He claimed he had gained clairvoyance and insight into life that all vegetation has been "endowed with sensitiveness." He said he was ashamed to speak the truth of his being a vegetable and that sane people considered him a lunacy-addled old codger. He asserted that plants and vegetables have feelings like humans and recoil at pain. How can one argue with Ichabod Artichoke? To bolster his claim, he noted the fact sunflowers turn their faces to the sun. He pleaded with the woodsman to no longer murder his kinsmen, the trees. He begged humanity to stop sinning with their eyes open. He asked that visitors not step on the grass, as they would injure his relatives. He asked all to acknowledge the living vegetables and leave them to their lives.

Impressions of the Passing Hour

This writing by "an ex-patient" mentioned random things that he as an "Uticanian" had casually observed or remembered while staying at the asylum. Nature was observed with admiration of the bespangled lawn of the asylum adorned with many yellow boys (dandelions), the soft summer breeze, the cedar shade where a rabbit made his home, the decayed hemlock on the hill that hosted a multitude of insects and the gay gilded lilies under the clouds of the heralded day. The writer also mentioned the love of "being odd" and the endless ticking of the asylum clocks but made the observation they were not keeping proper precise time. The writer recalled passing the time with other patients by inventing funny names, describing the physical descriptions of fellow patients. One was called a "copper kettle of boiling cider" and another who had "unmistakably massive proportions." The writer described the temperaments and afflictions of fellow patients yet neglected to describe their own. The writer finally mentioned ghosts, practical jokers of the mind, insanity being of "mediocrity" and how the patients are acting and playing the game of life to either stay in the asylum under the flag of insanity or carry the banner of being sane through the front gates in a return to society. The article ends with the writer asking, "Reader, are we happy now? Adieu now! Fork is the word."

Immensity of Motion and Animal Life in the Creation

In reading articles in the *Opal*, you come to realize that some of the passages are a little bizarre and ramblings of people not in their right minds; however, some are extremely academic, well written and insightful. There is no doubt from reading many of these articles that mental illness did not mean one lacked intelligence. The article written by D.S. on the motions of the planets was amazing considering the lack of scientific data in the mid-nineteenth century. Watching the celestials was limited to the strength of the telescopes at the time, yet D.S. made some amazing declarations on the movements of the planets and the universe. He wrote about the position of the sun and planets, their temperatures, their orbits and the movement of our solar system as part of the Milky Way Galaxy. He claimed that stars are of their own illumination and not reflective of our sun. He cited the illustrious Dr. Herschel as the discoverer of many of the facts in his article, including the position and movement of sunspots, the distance of planets, and temperatures on their surfaces. All this data is incredible considering the available science at the time. D.S. asserted that God had created all of it, and even though we are in his image, the almighty spread his creation vastly beyond the earth. D.S. even wrote of the microscope, beings invisible to the naked eye yet in their own universe the size of a head of a pin. The only part of the article where D.S. is off base is his claim that all planets contain alien life. He said it's a "very strong probability" and that there is "truth in the doctrine" based on the evidence by Dr. Herschel. It's fascinating to read people's theories on things we take for granted in our modern age.

Kingdom of the Fairies

One writer of the *Opal* told a story of walking the outer garden of the lunatic asylum and chancing upon a spiral ladder that was made of blue convolvulus vine that went down into the haunt, the chosen retreat of the kingdom of the fairies. She witnessed them hiding under the flowers and described the creatures as wearing little green jackets that hid them well among the flora. She said there were two kinds of fairies that were easily differentiated by the light emitted from their eyes. The evil fairies had a green light from their eyes that she considered to be from jealousy. The light from the eyes of the good fairies was transparent—so much so that a person under the influence of them was attracted to beauty and order. The fairies had blades of grass for swords that would rust under the midnight dew. The fairies used fireflies as their midnight lanterns. The writer stated that she witnessed a young girl under the spell of the beautifully dressed and adorned fairies who went and ate deadly nightshade then became deathly ill, yet the good fairies used their flapping wings to cool the young girl's brow until dawn came. She was cheered by a halo of goodness and then awoke to appreciation and love to the fairies. Afterward the young girl was affected differently by different flowers, and her soul was attracted to the elegance of the scent.

Public Amusement

In one editorial, the unknown writer lamented the fact the patients were bound to the asylum, especially when the summer sun hit the Mohawk Valley and everyone it seemed traveled to the lakes and streams for picnics and fun. The writer bemoaned not being able to enjoy the "pleasures of summer." Watering places are mentioned along with the activities of fishing, hunting, courting and other enjoyments. The editorial included Trenton Falls, Saratoga, Clifton, Niagara, Nahunt and other places hundreds of ladies and gentlemen, Sabbath schools, military companies and orphan asylums enjoyed, all accessible by rail. In our modern world, it's easy to jump in our automobiles and scramble to a nearby lake or pond, but back in the mid-nineteenth century, it was a grand adventure in which the patients at the Lunatic Asylum at Utica were banned from participating. It's funny to read how the author of this lamentation mentioned the vulgarity of the new country dancing being done and how the managers at the asylum let them leave the grounds, very briefly, in the winter, for a sleigh ride. Thus, being committed, the patients were held to the grounds for their care, their safety and the security of the general public. Still, the writer of this piece wanted to meet with "pigs, poultry and pretty country girls." They conclude by saying people should "excuse us from wailing from our prison-house."

The Erie and Chenango Canal

The opening of the Erie Canal created an industrial boom for cities that sat along the banks of the commerce-laden waterway. Utica became connected in the early nineteenth century and was considered the halfway point, making it a popular stopping place for travelers. Travelers marveled at the growth of Utica, but the most curious must have wondered what to make of the large asylum sitting upon the hill in West Utica. Within the 1859 volume 9 of the *Opal*, an anonymous writer mentioned the patients at the asylum being able to see the goods-laden boats floating down the Erie Canal. The writer said that the vessels were loaded with goods from the west like potatoes, potash, flour, shingles, staves, coal and wood. The writer called the ferry boats "silent ministers to the wants and comforts of the great cities that glide noiselessly past our windows like phantoms." There was a vast aggregate of wealth in taking goods to the markets. Utica also had the Chenango Canal, which operated from 1834 to 1878 and connected the Susquehanna River to the Erie Canal. These waterways made Utica an important city in the northeastern United States.

THE *OPAL* SPONSORS

For nine years, the *Opal* was able to sustain its expense by subscribers and local Utica businesses that paid to advertise in the monthly magazine. The price of subscription for one year was one dollar. An issue was published every month and generated revenue for the print shop. The following appeared on the last page of some of the issues in a plea for books, periodicals, money or subscriptions:

> *THE* OPAL
>
> *Commends itself to the generous and philanthropic, whose sympathies are with the unfortunate, and whose hearts are open to contribute to their relief.*
>
> *One great source of benefit and happiness to all of us, and especially to those whose residence here will, perhaps, be life-long, is the perusal of interesting books; but we are in a great measure deprived of the advantages derived from this source, since the State has made no appropriation for a Library for our use. One grand object in publishing the Opal is to extend a knowledge of our wants to a generous public who cannot but be interested in our welfare.*
>
> *From Authors, Publishers, and Booksellers, also from humane societies, churches, and private individuals, we shall be happy to receive contributions, either in subscriptions to the Opal, books or money; and if in money, we will apply it to the purchase of books they may direct; and if no direction is given, will expend it in adding to our library such books as will, in the judgment of the officers, be most proper and useful. All contributions will be promptly acknowledged in our pillars.*
>
> *TERMS—ONE DOLLAR PER ANNUM IN ADVANCE.*
>
> *Address, "The Opal, State Lunatic Asylum, Utica, N.Y."*

POETRY

The following selected poems were written by the patients at the Lunatic Asylum at Utica and published within the pages of the *Opal* from 1851 to 1860. Some of the spellings are incorrect and some words are obscure in today's life; however, these are best replicated exactly how they appeared over 150 years ago. These selected poems are ones that caught the fancy of the author or were deemed important as they apply to life in the asylum. These poems are not the complete works. Some of the poems are about animals, especially birds, while some poems comment on the fashion of the day and facial hair. Some of the poems portray the lonely life of the asylum while others embrace life. Some of these poems are what we would label as "politically incorrect" and are offensive, amateurish and shocking; however, they needed to be included to give you, dear reader, a sense of the world these patients were living in and society in the Mohawk Valley in the mid-nineteenth century. When you read these poems, think of the people who were placed in the asylum and the freedom of expression provided by the *Opal*. These show that people who were in the asylum had the intelligence and passion of poets.

Asylumia

by Anonymous

It is not wise, or always kind
To tell the workings of the mind,
To say, how father's apples grow,
Or how many boats the steamers tow;
Nor is it best to fill with prate
Most precious hours, with dull relate
Of trifling incidents of life
That show sometimes an ugly wife:
Or woes, or joys, or perfect bliss,
That hang suspended on a kiss,
Of gardens full of rosy bowers,
And walks mid castellated towers,
Nor rovers teeming with the pride
Of those who like a water ride---
It is not always wise to say
"How pleasant it is here to day."

Or look awhile for happy morrow,
Beams of joy for hope to borrow;

Or even when out on lovers' spark
To say who kisses in the dark---
There are so many threescore-ten
That tell us what we might have been,
There are so many broken leaves,
To think of them, my heart it grieves,
But oh! it is not here to pass,
Every sweet and black eyed lass,
Though she may cast an angry dart
That'll pierce the tenderness of the heart,
And cause a lingering dullish pain
That may lead one among the Insane;
And it is best to have good laws,
And sometimes to come to a pause.

The Early Dead

to Katie M --.

O! blessed are the early dead,
Who pass from earth in life's bright day,
ere sin their pure young hearts has led
Far from the paths of truth away,--

Ere yet their tender feet have trod
The thorny path of mortal life,
Safe with their Saviour and their God,
Forever freed from sin and strife.

'Tis true we sadly miss them here-
Their greeting voices, sunny smiles,
Their clinging confidence and love
Our weary, care-worn life beguiles.

But, Oh! we would not wish them back
From that bright world to earth again,

To walk with us the rugged track
Of disappointment, grief, and pain.

We know they're safe with Him who said,
"Bring little children unto me;"
His breast's the pillow for their head,
Their music angel's ministrelsy.

They are not lost, but gone before,
To rest far, far from grief and sin,
And wide is opened heaven's door
To let the little travelers in.

Thrice blessed are the early dead,
And though the bud opes not on earth,
'Twill bloom in heaven, and lustre shed
On flowers of celestial birth.

Then let us never more repine
When death shall lay our loved ones low;
God takes them to a fairer clime,
To purer bliss than mortals know.

Evening Lights at Asylumia

By C.

All things my lofty window-seat surrounding
To-night in wakeful vision meet my eye--
The town, the valley, and the far hills bounding
My realms of earth and sky.

Above, the star hosts in unstayed confession
Of their Creator, and the planets' bright,
Far-swinging censers throng the grand procession
Toward the Infinite.

The New York State Lunatic Asylum

Beneath, the city, by the dim night tapers
That point the chambers of its quiet rest,
And girt with spectral walls of fleecy vapors,
Reared on the waters' breast;

From whence the passing boat-lamps feebly glimmer,
In their slow orbit through the misty space;
And comet-lights rush forth in startling shimmer
Along the railway's trace.

On these long gazing, while the dreamy curtain
Of night o'er Summer's charms is slowly drawn,
The starry scene begins to grow uncertain,
And other lights to dawn.

The light of childhood's years, in pureness beaming
The far horizon of my dream of life,
Sheds o'er my soul a heavenly radiance, seeming
With spirit memories rife.

And from my longed-for home's dear fireside, nearer
And warmer issuing, the sweet visions fall;
With glowing love-light from one face, O dearer,
Dearer to me than all!

Thus, memory-lit, my heart's fond vigil keeping,
Till comes again that deep, mysterious gloom,
Each gleam of faith and hope in blackness steeping,
I seek my lonely room.

My soul! the splendors of the nightly azure,
The radiant affluence of the sleeping earth,
Thy present mercies, and the past's bright treasure:--
Why still thy rayless dearth?

O Thou! who shinest in divine effulgence,
Th' unfailing source of universal light!
My feeble, doubting prayers yet grant indulgence;
Dispel my weary night!

Death

By Anonymous

Why call death fearful! why does a thrill
Pass over us when His dread name we hear?
Why does the heart leap up, and then be still,
And the thick breath come fast with trembling fear?
There is no cause for terror, and the voice,
If heard aright will make the heart rejoice.

We hear it in the storm that rends the sky,
We hear it in the low wind's sadden'd tone,
It speaks to us in summer evening's sigh,
And in our own sad hearts when grieved and lone.
It calls to us among the leaves and flowers,
We hear it in the quickly passing hours.

In youth, in manhood, in old age it comes;
In joy, in sorrow, still it's voice we hear,
Wherever we may be, abroad, at home,
Yet still that certain, low, hush'd tone is there,
It tells in the breeze that sweeps the grass
Fading its freshness, that we too must pass.

Is it not pleasant? When afar we roam,
Away from kindred souls in distant lands,
How sweet each record we receive from home;
Each precious letter traced by gentle hands;
Death is the message that our Father sends,
To call us to our home, and absent friends.

To Our Pharmacopolists

By Etta Floyd

I know that so weary, my friends, you must be,
You wish that from powders and pills you were free.
Your olfactories sure might well ask for release,
From all the unwelcome perfumes that increase.

Those opiates strong must inertness oft cause,
Not strange would it be should you oft make a pause,
But then you've enough to enliven you too,
So fear not that harm can ever ensue.

Not scarce are your tinctures and essences good,
That long have the trial of ill ones withstood;
Fine extracts and lotions that benefit some,
And aids for the deaf, if not the dumb.

Now if you've the rare, and most wonderful art.
To light the "dark" mind, or heal the SICK HEART,
Do just persevere in oft showing your skill,
And plenty of dollars your purses shall fill.

We'll hope that for all the relief you bestow,
The choiciest of blessings may long overflow,
And when kindly fortune shall send you a wife,
She'll ever be known as the joy of your life.

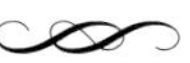

To Dr. G- -y

By Anonymous

Who is the being bright and kind
That comes to reason's darkened mind

And brings a sweet and blessed ray?
It is our own kind Dr. G- -y.

Who charms away the dismal mood
With precepts ever wise and good?
Ah! Words of consolation, they
Fall from the lips of Dr. G- -y.

His face benevolent and kind,
Bespeaks the feelings of his mind.
What drives the clouds of fear away?
'Tis the glad smile of Dr. G- -y.

Oh Gratitude! The world's too cold,
To express the feelings all untold,
That rush into the mind each day,
When we think of thee, kind Dr. G- -y.

How can I leave a theme so full,
Of all that's bright and beautiful?
Accept this warm and heartfelt lay,
And blessings fall on Dr. G- -y.

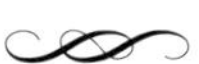

Thoughts

Suggested by seeing the sun suddenly shining through my asylum room after a cloudy day

Was it a sunbeam came to cheer
This troubled soul of mine?
Was it a ray from heaven above,
So thrilling—so divine?

Was it a beam of peace and love
Came to this wretched, wand'ring heart?
Was it a ray of God's own truth,
To bid my woes and fears depart?

Was it a flood of light divine,
That came to wash my sins away?
Through Jesus' blood to make me clean,
And open up eternal day?

Yes! Once he cleansed this sinful heart,
Spoke peace and comfort to the soul;
Bade fear and misery depart,
And made the hopeless sinner whole!

Yes! He redeemed me from the gloom,
The night and darkness of despair,
Averted then the threatening doom
Which hung its fearful shadows there.

He bade me sing anew his praise,
His grace and wondrous love repeat,
His justice see in all His ways;
He led me to the mercy seat.

Thou savedst me, Lord, by wondrous grace.
To thee, through Christ, my life is given,
Thou said'st "I'll never hide my face"*
That promise to my heart is heaven.
*Ezekiel 34.29
Nov. 28, 1852

To the Asylum Band

By Anonymous

Oh! Come and play that strain once more
That I so dearly love;
'Twas listened to in days of yore
By some that dwell above.

Oh! Come and play - - and come again,
Then I will cease to grieve;
I never heard a sweeter strain
Than that I heard last eve.

Oh! Come and play it o'er and o'er,
It ne'er will cease to charm;
The aching heart still pants for more,
For such it ne'er can harm.

Oh! Come, ye merry band, and play
My fav'rite tune once more; --
Come 'neath the moon's soft, silvery ray
Come closer to the door.

Oh! Come again to us and play
Until the clock chimes eleven;
And thus, we all will hope to meet
This merry band in Heaven.

I Dreamed I Was a Fairy

By Anonymous

Yes, I lived in halls of lovely pearl,
With rainbow colors it was inlaid,
I sat on a throne of rare beauty,
It was of diamonds and coral made.

And Fairies dressed in green, and gold,
Merrily flitted past my throne,
I spoke to them, they headed not,
But soon did leave me all alone.

The distant sound of music,
At length did reach my ear,

The gentle dashing of waters
Told there was a fountain near.

But then I awoke,
For somebody to me spoke,
Saying, if the ladies don't get up,
They must go to bed right after sup.

Riding on a Rail

By Ned Sanders

From Auburn jail, as you shall know,
Where "Freemen rolled" long ago,
Ned Sanders started, in the snow,
For home, by rail-rode rapidly.

Kind words were those, by Norman said:
"Is any body with you, Ned,
To keep your nose clean—save your head
From getting crazed, at Auburn city?"

'Twas kind in Miller—kind in White,
To bind Ned Sanders fast and tight;
Such is the "common law"—it's right,
And Sanders heeds it reverently.

Ned Sanders "saw another sight,"
When his chains clanked at deed at night,
Provoking madness, in her might,
To join their dev'lish deviltry!

Ned's fetters gall'd his shins and pride;
Through all their dev'lish rail-road ride,
Chain'd, as he was, close by his side
Of Fashion's proud gentility.

Three hundred fifty miles or more,
Ned Sanders rode in sweat and gore,
Ere he was landed at his door,
In madness, raving fearfully!

Long weeks Ned passed quite crazily,
And when he saw the dawn of day,
He found himself at Utica,
Well used, and treated sensibly!

Sounds Heard in the Asylum at Night

By S.H.B.

Shattering strings—shattering strings!
Mournful tones ye utter now;
Through the night your discord rings,
Jarring on my fever'd brow.
Oh, what noble, heavenly harps,
Here unstrung and useless lie!
Some, perchance, will ne'er ring true,
'Till eternity!

Then, those chords, if once attun'd
To the blessed Savior's praise,
Though they ne'er again on earth
Aught but notes discordant raise,

Shall awake with rapturous swell,
When that "new song" shall be given—
Oh, these harps of "thousand strings"
Will ring out true in Heaven!

The "smiling face" will yet beam out
From this "frowning Providence;"
The "Silver lining" yet to be seen

To the cloud now darkling thence:
All that's dim be clear as day,
Things mysterious, made plain;
Shattering strings, -- shattering strings,
When ye're tuned again!

Dark Days

by Etta Floyd

In vain we look for brighter days,
The sun still recreant proves, --
Not one stray beam around us plays,
As onward still he moves.

Why is it that he hath withdrawn
His genial, cheering light,
And on each new successive morn
No scene we find this bright?

Each day the rain comes falling fast--
Eolus stronger grows--
While earth with darkness is o'ercast
Till day doth on it close.

At times it something brighter seems,
And hope then quickly springs,
But ah! short-lived these sudden gleams,
And dull despair still clings.

What shall we do to woo once more
The long-lost orb of day--
Effulgence o'er the earth to pour,
And still his charms display?

What lack there is of sun some tell
By smiles must be supplied--
That these the darkness will dispel,
And make hours faster glide.

"Suffer On."

By Cecelia

Suffering is the "bud of glory,"
Ere it burst the mental gloom;
Weeping is the dewy story,
Till the heart-felt influence come;

Every blade is tipp'd with diamonds,
Every channel grace hath wet,
Till the "King of Glory" summons
Faith's loud-calling "minaret."

Symphony of angel music,
Every sigh from heaven's acclaim;
Louder strikes the note beatific
For a care-worn creature's frame.

Sacrifice is worth the spending, --
'Tis pure incense to the "All-wise;"
With such gifts the alter bending,
Ecstatic Hope re-gains the prize.

Languishing, distress'd, or weary,
Disease's the cordial for thy soul;
Would'atthon not sicken for Heaven's glory?
Final possession is the goal!

Lines

By Anonymous

"We need more than all other comforts, the presence and retaining influence of intelligent and pure-minded women. Cannot you send us Californians, some of your many lovely Yankee girls."

Extract of a letter.

Oh ladies fair! A pleading voice
Comes daily o'er the waters,
List to the cry dear Empire maids,
And Pennsylvania's daughters,
Then tell it to the Buckeye girls,
And the tall Hoosier lasses
Yes send it by the telegraph,
Thro' vales and rocky passes.

Proclaim it to the Yankee belles
Aye! Keep the ball in motion
And soon we'll send a precious freight,
Swift speeding o'er the ocean,
In California's countless mines
The yellow ore is shining,
But in her thousand lonely homes
Strong manly hearts are pining.

When wearied with the daily task,
No looming welcome greets them,
No sunny smile, or gentle face,
At their own threshold meets them:
No soft hand bathes the aching head,
Or smoothes the downy pillow,
Alas! No tender wives have they
And so the wear the willow.

Then Susy, Mary, Lizzie, Kate.
Go cheer the heart-sick fellows

Who dig for gold, and seek for wealth
Far o'er the bounding billows;
Their mourning shall be turned to joy
Their sighs, to songs of gladness,
For woman's presence ever proves
The antidote for sadness.

Soliloquy

By a Blind Boy Who Fancied He Would See on the Fourth of July

Oh, Mother, dear Mother,
When shall I see?
When the Fourth of July
Brings its morning to me!

To all free men it comes
In its proudest array;
For the Fourth of July
Is a Nation's birth-day.

Oh Mother, dear Mother,
When shall I see?
When the Fourth of July
Brings its Freedom to me!

Then I'll whisper in accents,
So tuneful and clear!
And none but my Mother,
Their import shall hear.

Mother, dear Mother!
When I shall see--
That morning of light,
Brings deliverance to thee.*

E'en now, dearest Mother,
A blest reverie near,
Comes auspicious of hope,
For that light of the year.

And then, dearest Mother!
Oh then should I see.
I'll whisper thee only,
That light's come to me.

Soft voices awaken
The hope, I shall see
When the Fourth of July
Brings its morning to me.

**The Mother of the Blind Boy suffered a voluntary confinement of one year with him in a darkened room.*

Pills vs Bleeding

By A.M.A.

My folks one day thought I was sick,
And for a Doctor they did speak,
So then as sure as I'm alive,
A great big quack did soon arrive.

With whiskers long, and eyes quite black,
Thinks I old fellow you I'll sack;
He talked of this and then of that,
While in my room sedate he sat.

I thought he'd nothing do but talk,
And out my room would quickly walk.
He soon commenced his operations
In spite of all my remonstrations

A box of pills were in his hand,
Which made my hair on end to stand,
These are for you said he to me,
And from all pain they'll set you free.

So pills I took, both black and blue,
But still no good they seemed to do,
For I grew still more sick and sore,
While pills each day I took a score.

Till at last I out of patience got,
And from the pills relief I sought;
Still in spite of all I could do
They crammed them down me not a few.

The doctor now at once did see
That pills were not the thing for me.
Some other means I'll have to try,
Or else this man will surely die.

Next day he came me for to bleed,
Although of blood I stood in need,
So out it came, the shining lance,
Oh then how I did jump and dance.

But three strong men of me took hold,
Which I did think was very bold,
They held me firm, they held me fast,
Till doctor he got through at last.

But still I did no better get,
Which made the Doctor scold and fret,
Pills and bleeding were all in vain,
To take away this awful pain.

Said he to me your very ill,
So now prepare to make your will,
And for another world make ready,
For there you know you must be steady.

But yet my friends did not believe,
That I soon this world would leave,
So off they went for Doctor S.
Who came and found me in distress.

He thought that I would soon get well,
If he could Doctor me a spell,
To work he went with all his might,
And wrapped me in a blanket tight.

To steam me now he did begin,
Which I did think was quite a sin,
What can he mean by this thought I,
He surely wants to have me die.

Hot tea he gave me quite enough,
How I did hate that nasty stuff,
It made me feel so very bad,
I really thought I would go mad.

The Doctors all did what they could,
Although they did but little good,
To cure the body and the mind,
A remedy they could not find.

So when their skill was put to test,
And each had tried to do his best,
They said no help there was for me,
For I a sufferer must be.

Meanwhile my friends were all distracted
To see the way in which I acted;
To Utica they brought me then,
And left me with the crazy men.

I have been here six months and more,
And feel as well as ever before.
Now glad am I the news to tell,
That I at last have got quite well.

The Time When I Would Die

By Anonymous

Oh, let me mid the smiles of May
Bid earth farewell, and pass away!
When the last ray of sunset hour
Still lingers on each bud and flower,
Then let me die!

When Winter's stern and icy chain,
Has burst, and Spring has come again;
When all the fields are rob'd in green,
And naught but beauty can be seen,
Then let me die!

Though far the sweetest time to live,
When sweet May flowers their odors give,
"Tis then my spirit fain would fly
To brighter realms above the sky,
Then let me die!

Ere the bright hopes of youth are past,
Full many a heart with sorrows cast;
But, when assur'd the Savior's near,
Then let me go, I have naught to fear.
'Tis sweet to die!

April—Day in the Asylum

By Anonymous

April first was a merry day,
For wit and folly both had play,
And each did with the other vie,
Which should excel in foolery,

Perhaps it were not well or meet,
Our morning fooleries to repeat;
The dinner too was soon passed by,
Without much noise, or hue and cry.

But when the bell with summons shrill,
The supper table 'gan to fill;
A goodly row of deep tureens,
With covers close, formed quite a screen

Between the sides, and promise made,
That something *"nice"* within was laid.
Thiose nearest them, with eager wish,
The covers lifted, neither fish,

Nor fowl, nor ought that could,
A substitute, appear for food,
Were visible, but empty dishes,
Soon left us nought but empty wishes.

"The Faculty" were forthwith called,
And dishes again overhauled,
To say if in their wise opinion,
The supper would *"do without an onion."*

But whether fear that rats or mice,
Were snugly covered there so nice,
Or what restrained them, nought could make
Them, the slight service undertake

To lift the covers, and explore
The mysteries, which they covered o'er:
So 'stead of cakes, we had some fun,
Nor with the day-light was it done;

For spite of warning to take care,
The lamps, well filled with vinegar,
Would *"patience of Job"* require,
Nought could induce them to take fire:

And burned fingers were *"the go,"*
And whispers quick of *"now you know,"*
But don't you tell, for that will spare
"Attempts, in which the all must share."

And when that laugh, had well gone by,
And *"Bed Time Ladies"* was the cry,
You'd find the broom in gown and cap,
Prepared with you to take a nap.

But all the doings to declare,
Would take more time, than we've to spare,
And could you have but seen the half,
You surely could not choose, but laugh.

And now against advice, if you
Will still persist, to read this through,
"Do you guv it up" that you have been
In April Fooling taken in?

Then don't complain that this is dull,
But own, that you're an April fool.

Death

By Matty

The king of terrors spreads his sway,
And singles out his fallen prey;
The old and young, the rich and poor,
Bow at his rod and are no more.

His presence's fear'd with dread by all,
Both high and low, - both great and small;
With ne repsect to wealth or name
He slays his thousands, still the same.

The widow's tears, - he heeds them not,
The orphan's moan, - by him's forgot;
The king upon his throne, likewise
Yields to his grasp, no more to rise.

The hope of man he doth destroy,
And withers all his earthly joy;
The dying one, - struggling for breath,
Falls in the icy arms of death.

His ruthless hand is ever near,
We know not when he will appear;
At morn, at midnight, or at noon,
We may be summon'd to the tomb.

Oh, Lord! Renew this heart of mine, -
Make it pure and wholly thine;
When I resign this fleeting breath,
May I with pleasure, welcome death.

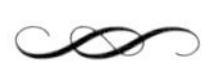

A Patient's Farewell to the Asylum

By S.R.B.

(The following "farewell" was read in the course of the lecture on Practical Insanity, delivered here by a patient, on the evening of Pinel's birthday, April 11th, 1856. If the composition and measure are not of the smoothest kind, they are the breathings of a grateful spirit.)

'Twas on the fifteenth day of December last,
That cold and stormy day,
I left my wife and family
In trouble and dismay.

I had no hopes of this vain world,
Nor in eternity;
My life was but a dreary dream,
And all was lost to me.

My friends around me did convene
To comfort and console,
But all they said or did for me
I felt like Uncle Job of old.

'Twas then I came to the Asylum,
Not thinking long to stay,
But they closed the doors and locked me in,
To pass my time in gloom away.

When I'd been there a week or two,
Not knowing what to do,
Bright light appeared to me by day,
And swept my gloomy thoughts away.

'Twas then my mind returned to me,
My troubles passed away;
I felt that sympathy again
I hope will with me stay.

For others I could sympathize
Whom in trouble I did see,

And call on God, with all my heart.
To pass their troubles all away.

And now, my friends, to one and all,
Who longer have to stay,
May you be blessed with good success,
And shortly get away.

Now gents and ladies, all farewell,
My respects to you I pay;
With feeling heart I now depart,
And leave you here to sing and pray.

Good luck unto our patients all,
And officers likewise;
We're in hopes of returning home again
To our sweethearts and our wives.
Chorus. —To our sweethearts and our wives, brave boys!

John P. Gray, MD (1854–1886)

Dr. John Gray took over supervision of the asylum after the death of Dr. Benedict. He was born in 1925 in Half Moon, Pennsylvania. His lengthy career was one of brilliant administration. He received his degree from the University of Pennsylvania in 1848 and was placed on the staff at the Lunatic Asylum at Utica in 1850 and stayed there for the rest of his professional life. Dr. Gray was a brilliant and respected man who was nationally revered in the world of mental illness, its diagnosis and treatment. He was president of the Oneida County Medical Society in 1872 and the New York State Medical Society in 1884.

Dr. Gray had a philosophy of medical care to insane patients that would be on par with the best medical hospitals. Diet, patient care and comfortable conditions were his watch words. Although he did continue to use the Utica crib, he preferred to let rambunctious patients roam free in a day room, feeling this methodology had a better effect on the patients. The great fires of the asylum occurred under his watch on July 14 and 18, 1857. One caused loss of life and significant damage. After the fires, many donations came

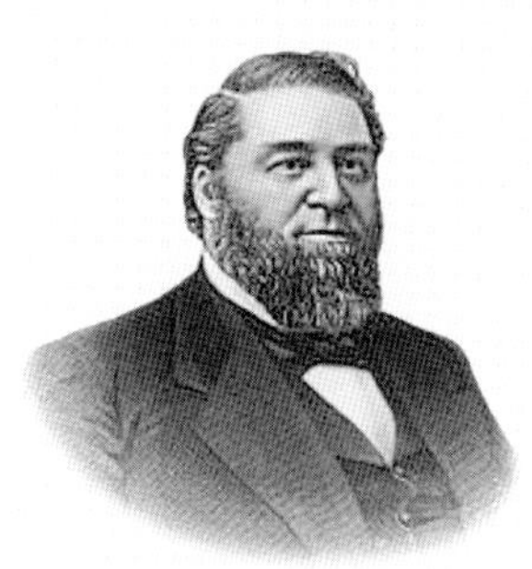

Dr. John Gray, Old Main superintendent (1854–1886). *New York State Archives.*

in to replace lost items. Leaders in Utica paid for a new organ for the chapel. All sorts of new firefighting equipment was purchased, including a hose house, hose carts, hoses, a steam fire pump, ladders and other mechanical equipment. The other item changed after the fire was the removal of the asylum gas house. The asylum contracted with the Utica Gas Company to supply the institution with gas light. By 1860, the asylum was hosting an average of 516 patients. The New York State legislature appropriated $20,000 in 1857 for a structure to be built in Auburn to house the criminally insane. Dr. Gray opposed the Willard Act, passed on April 5, 1865, as the law mandated a separation of the most chronically ill mental patients. Dr. Gray, and many physicians, opposed this separation, as it was against the philosophy of Dr. Brigham, for whom Dr. Gray had great admiration. The law resulted in the Willard Asylum, which was built in 1869 to house the "chronic insane." With 1,500 beds, Willard was now the largest asylum in the country, as it was filled with the poor and mentally ill from almshouses all around New York State and even some patients of Utica.

Dr. Gray added innovations like detailed record keeping on patients' symptoms and results of autopsies. He implemented photography and photomicrography in conjunction with pathological work. Dr. Gray edited the *American Journal of Insanity* and published his results of these tests and procedures, garnering him worldwide respect. Dr. Gray oversaw the construction of the stone-pillared front entrance and the erection of the iron fence on the York Street side of the property. The fencing was donated from the Capital Park in Albany by the legislature. It also provided $3,000 to transport and erect the fencing. In 1875, after the installation of the iron fence, brand-new cast-iron radiators were installed along with a new heating system designed by the asylum engineer Joseph Graham. It came to be known as the Utica Pattern and was copied by other national asylums. In 1874, Dr. Gray oversaw the construction of a small hospital for ill and pregnant women. In 1879, day rooms and sunrooms were added for patient comfort.

In 1885, new additions were added to house disturbed patients, but a huge, hazardous crack in the northwestern wall of the main building was discovered. It had been built on quicksand. The legislature appropriated

$20,000 to fix the problem, and the cracked corner was propped up by steel girders and all the quicksand removed. A new reinforced wall was built and new fill placed in the area. By this time, Utica was growing as an industrial city and encroaching on the borders of the asylum, yet the two-hundred-acre farm was still operational and all the workshops busy and making money for the asylum. The asylum entertainment hall, or stage, from September to April, hosted plays, musical performances, lectures and other amusements twice a week. The patients were still putting on many performances, but the stage was small and on the fifth floor, so Dr. Gray asked for appropriations to construct a new hall. The asylum didn't have the huge tourist and visitor numbers from the 1850s but still reported one thousand visitors a month in 1886.

Dr. Gray was said to be highly sociable and required his young physician assistants to be proper gentlemen and in the Utica public eye. The doctor was called to Washington, D.C., as expert witness to the trial of Charles Guiteau, who assassinated President Garfield. He was to testify on the sanity of the assassin. Guiteau was found guilty and executed on June 30, 1882. When Dr. Gray returned, he was almost killed by an angry man over his testifying. Dr. Gray was sitting in his office with his son and a staff physician when Henry Remshaw of Utica stormed in, leveled his pistol and fired. Dr. Gray turned his head and received a bullet wound across his nose; the projectile entered under his eye and became embedded in the wall of his face. The wound did not kill Dr. Gray. It was discovered that Remshaw was mentally ill but had never been committed to the asylum. The man was deranged and was committed to the Auburn asylum for the criminally insane.

Dr. Gray was diagnosed with Bright's disease and took a sabbatical in February 1886 down south to improve his health. He took a trip abroad to seek a cure. He returned to his duties at the asylum in October but passed away from the disease on November 27, 1886. Dr. John Perdue Gray had been the asylum superintendent for thirty-two years.

The Nursing School

Once again, Utica would be at the forefront of innovation and improvement in patient care by the creation of a nursing school. Dr. Gray made an important decision in 1883, creating a plan by which asylum attendants

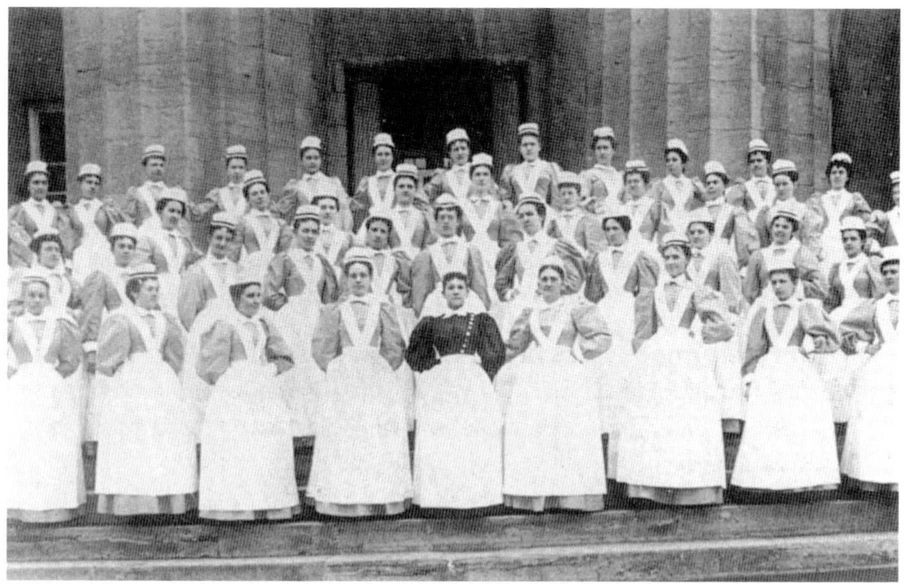

The asylum's School of Nursing students posing on the front steps. *New York State Archives.*

and nurses would be educated to enhance services to the patients. Teaching plans and lectures by the medical staff began in the asylum. The topics included anatomy, physiology, hygiene, diet and general patient care. The nursing school would expand under Dr. Gray's successor, Dr. Alder Blumer, with 59 nurses receiving a certified diploma for the first time in 1892. They would have to pass written and oral exams. There would be no graduation ceremony for the nurses until 1909. Old Main would continue to educate and graduate nurses from the two-year program until 1922, when the Utica State Hospital School of Nursing merged with Faxton, St. Elizabeth and St. Luke's Hospitals to create one centralized school of nursing. By this time, the school had 466 graduates. Marcy State Hospital began a school of nursing in the late 1940s, with nurses being sent to Utica College for nursing programs in 1950. The New York State Office of Mental Hygiene started to phase out the schools of nursing, with the last nursing class of Utica State Hospital graduating in May 1975. The combined schools of nursing had educated nurses for eighty-six years, graduating a total of 1,472.

The Great Fire

One of the most dramatic, traumatic and scariest events in the history of the asylum was the great fire of July 14, then a smaller barn fire on July 18, both in 1857. At 7:00 a.m. on July 14, a fire was discovered in the middle part of Old Main. West Utica engine no. 7 responded and found that the only water immediately available was from a well at the rear of the asylum. The only other water was from the Erie Canal, which was two thousand feet from the building and down a hill. The Utica Fire Department was able to get a single stream from the well and had to carry it to the roof to pour down on the fire.

The *Journal* newspaper from Lowville, New York, wrote at the time:

> *The most fearful feature of the scene was the awful cry of the lunatics 500 to 600 in number who were inmates of the building. The men, who were kept in the right hand building, were relatively quiet but the screams and antics of the females in the left hand building, were appalling. The larger portion of ladies uttered heart rendering cries for relief, many howled prayers at the tops of their voices, while others made the air crazy with unintelligible songs. Many of the females were removed and taken to a grove behind the asylum.*

Lines of men, staff members and the Utica firefighters formed a bucket brigade on the third floor to dump water on the fire to keep it from spreading to the wings. It descended from the attic, where it had started, through the floors to the basement. In saving the asylum furniture, several men were burned and severely injured. Dr. Rose, of the asylum, was rescuing furniture when a large piece of burning ceiling plaster and wood came down upon his head and killed him. Utica firefighter William Cressford also died when burning timbers fell on him. It was now 11:00 a.m., and the New York Mills and Whitesboro Fire Departments showed up just in time, as the well had run dry. They were able to get a stream of water from the Erie Canal. The day was hot and humid, and the large fire was causing many firefighters to drop from heat exhaustion. A call was sent out to Rome, Herkimer and Little Falls Fire Departments. Rome firemen placed their equipment on a train car and were able to arrive at the burning asylum in twenty-eight minutes. A train car also delivered the Little Falls and Herkimer equipment right after. The extra firefighters were able to get a second water stream from the Erie Canal.

During the fire, Deputy Sheriff Klinek and his deputies arrived, along with the local Citizens Corps, German Rifles and local artilleries. They did not fight the fire but formed a circle around Old Main. Their mission was to keep asylum patients from escaping and also protect the asylum and its contents from possible looters. Utica factories closed early, and tradesmen, clerks, mechanics and apprentices arrived in droves to assist the firefighters, as many had collapsed from the heat. The fire was finally extinguished at 3:00 p.m. None of the asylum patients were injured, but four more firefighters were severely burned when a flaming wall fell on them. They survived their injuries. The patients were able to sleep in their beds that night, as the wings had been saved and had no smoke or fire damage. In the middle building, the chapel, some patient sitting rooms, the dining room and the living room were lost.

Four days later, another fire hit the asylum complex when the barn was discovered ablaze. It was extinguished, and nobody was hurt or killed. One of the asylum staff caught William Speirs in the woods nearby hysterical with laughter. Speirs was a former patient of the asylum who upon release had been hired as an employee. Dr. Gray and other doctors and staff of the asylum questioned Speirs, and he was arrested and taken to the Oneida County Jail. The *New York Daily Tribune* wrote an editorial in which it criticized the asylum leadership for releasing Speirs. He had been a patient for many years before being released and given work at the asylum. Speirs had his keys taken away by Dr. Gray, so he decided to set fires out of retaliation. The newspaper revealed that Speirs had been an arsonist down in New York City and was incarcerated in the Blackwell's Island Asylum. Eventually, he was tried and sent to the asylum in Utica. The newspaper asked how a man could be cured when his disposition was to set fires upon the slightest provocation. It said that keeping Speirs deemed insane would have cost less than the damage his arson caused to a state asylum. The Lunatic Asylum at Utica responded to the criticism with an editorial response in which it stated, "The helpless fellow-creatures within our walls are under our care and the fire had caused a thrill of horror to every heart."

Dr. Gray testified in front of Judges Bacon, Denio and Root, Dr. Dering and the board of managers regarding the arsonist. He said that Speirs came to the asylum on January 14, 1850, and had previously been a patient at Blackwell's Island for eleven months for arson. He had been deranged and deemed insane. He was released as cured on February 1, 1856, and soon started to work at the asylum, as he was well liked by the entire staff. They said he was industrious, careful and thoughtful. He worked in the dining room and print shop. After a while, he became a handyman and received keys and full access to the asylum. Just before the fires, Dr. Gray took Speirs's keys away as punishment for using foul language. The man was penitent, so the keys were returned, but the mental arson rage had been lit. Speirs simmered underneath at being treated in what he perceived as a bad manner.

Speirs was put on trial and testified that he had started the fire in the middle structure attic of Old Main by lighting three piles of light wood and papers. He set the fires with candles. Five days later, he set the fire in the barn by using a match on a pile of dry hay. When asked why he did it, Speirs said Dr. Gray had taken his keys. Dr. Gray later admitted he had been wrong for giving Speirs keys. The arsonist was found guilty and committed to the Lunatic Asylum at Utica for the rest of his life. The damage was severe, and even conservative estimates at the time had it around $25,000. The asylum would be fixed and continue with patient care.

ARSONIST ON THE RUN

Although William Speirs had been arrested, charged, convicted and committed for the arson at the asylum, the August 1857 issue of the *Opal*, vol. 7, issue no. 8, printed a confessional letter from a patient identified only as H.S. who claimed to not only have set the fires but also chronicled and detailed his escape and the details of his days on the run. H.S. claimed to have run away from the asylum once before and lived on his ingenuity, wits and grit. He allegedly lasted three and a half years on the run and traveled three hundred miles before being captured and placed back in the asylum. H.S. said he started the fire and watched it for a bit before saving some books, including a Washington primer. He set off from Utica with two cents and a cracker and a half. He would stop at a tavern in the city, drank his two cents' worth of beer, begged some tobacco then went to the Erie Canal and commenced to walk the estimated one hundred miles to Albany. He had neither a coat nor a vest and found the day hot. The escapee made it twenty-three miles before sitting down on the hard ground, eating his crackers and drinking a little whiskey that he had been able to beg from passersby. He felt he had sunstroke but walked until dark then lay down on hard sod without a blanket and slept until 1:00 a.m. He got up stiff and sore and vulnerable to death. He paused for a moment, looked up to the heavens and sang, "Twinkle Twinkle Little Star." He moved on. He found a house along the way and was unable to beg anything and left with dogs barking at his heels.

The following day he came upon a farmhouse, and the kind residents gave him a large chunk of bread, butter, a slab of pork and water. They gave him some tobacco. He thanked them and moved along.

H.S. walked twenty miles that hot July day and stopped to bathe in the Mohawk River. He slept on the hard ground of a field and woke again at 1:00 a.m. and started off. He came to a town that had more than a few people and hid himself in the rear of a buggy, where he slept until a pack of dogs barking roused him. He petted the dogs and then made away until he found train tracks. He walked along and begged everywhere yet was unable to obtain anything. He came upon Amsterdam and tried to get a job as a printer and was turned away. He was able to get handy work and made five cents. He purchased some crackers and a glass of brandy. He walked on another twenty miles, where he met a person he described as a "darkie" who had a vicious dog that he had to fend off. He made his way to Schenectady, where he ate lemon peels, orange peels, cocoa nuts and a head of a herring. He tried to get a job in the city and couldn't but was able to acquire some crackers that he ate while watching a circus parade go down the main road.

After some crackers and cheese, H.S. walked fifteen more miles before bathing in the river and sleeping next to the canal. He walked again and came to a cottage, where he drank whiskey, smoked a pipe with the owner and danced a jig to a fiddle. He shook hands with the owner and moved on. He was farther down the road when a man on a horse came by and told him he had to watch where he was resting or he'd get run over and killed. H.S. walked off the path and slept in a barn in a hay-strewn stall next to a horse. He woke up in the morning and found cherries and raspberries. He picked as much as he could hold in his shirt and sat in the shade of an oak tree and ate them all. It was then that he realized he was only three miles from Albany. He yelled out "Yoicks!" with joy and zest. He was able to get a ride in a buggy the last leg of his journey and was overjoyed at making the capital. He drank some whiskey and saluted himself. He was able to beg twenty-two cents and a half penny and used the money to purchase oysters, ale and cigars. H.S. nearly got into a fight with a group of four men then went on to sleep on a sidewalk. A man of authority woke him and escorted him to what was referred to as a "station house," something like a place for the poor to sleep. He had a wonderful rest on a bed. He woke and found a day job and made enough to buy a beefsteak dinner and whiskey.

He decided to move on from Albany and took off all his clothes, washed them in a river and hung them on the branches of a tree. He was swimming naked when a group of boys and girls came along and teased him. He chuckled and then nearly drowned. He waited for them to leave before getting dressed in his damp clothes and moving on. The summer heat dried his clothes, and they stayed that way until the rain from a violent thunderstorm wet him. He'd been asleep on a sand bar next to the river when the lightning woke him. He heard music. It was away from the canal, so he walked toward the sound and came upon a pub with people playing bagpipes inside. He was welcomed and danced a jig and drank whiskey. He was able to share a bed with three other men and slept well until one kicked him in the shin. He tried in vain to get a job, as he wanted to pay for passage to New York City, but was unable. He was finally arrested and brought to an almshouse, where they gave him bread and cheese. In the morning, he got oyster stew and hot black coffee. They placed him in a railroad car, and he was returned to the asylum, where he saw the charred remains of the fire he had confessed to setting. He had been away for eleven days. When asked how he felt, H.S. smiled and said, "Jolly!"

This story could be the product of the imagination of William Speirs, as he had been arrested right after the barn fire when caught laughing in the woods while watching the second fire. He, at the time of the fires, had been deemed sane and was working at the asylum. After his trial for arson, he was recommitted to the Lunatic Asylum at Utica. Either the asylum management, staff and newspapers covered up his escape to keep the public from panic, or the escape story is just another part of his mania. Or it's a fictionalized account from the mysterious H.S.

Visitors

In the nineteenth century, as asylums were being built, for the first time in the history of our country, people afflicted with mental illness were collected at one place. According to Benjamin Reiss, author of the book *Theaters of Madness*, the Lunatic Asylum at Utica was attracting 2,700 visitors per year from 1843 to 1853, and this outpaced some of the best parks and attractions in the country. Dr. Brigham started the practice of admitting the public in order to show that the moral treatment was working along with the large taxpayer expense that had gone into the building of Old Main. In later years, visitors would be limited to doctors, visiting dignitaries, families and friends, as the spectacle had begun to be criticized. Over the years, there were visits by President Millard Fillmore, the New York State legislature, Dorothea Dix and many world-renowned physicians from asylums wanting to see the success of Old Main to replicate in their own facilities.

Form 126–Adm.

State of New York—Utica State Hospital

Permission is granted

M. A. Graff

to be absent from the Hospital

until 12 P m. Date Dec. 24

Returned .... m.

.... Nightwatch

F. C. Smith Per— M. A. G. Supervisor

Patient Christmas Eve pass from the nineteenth century. *Courtesy Dennis Webster.*

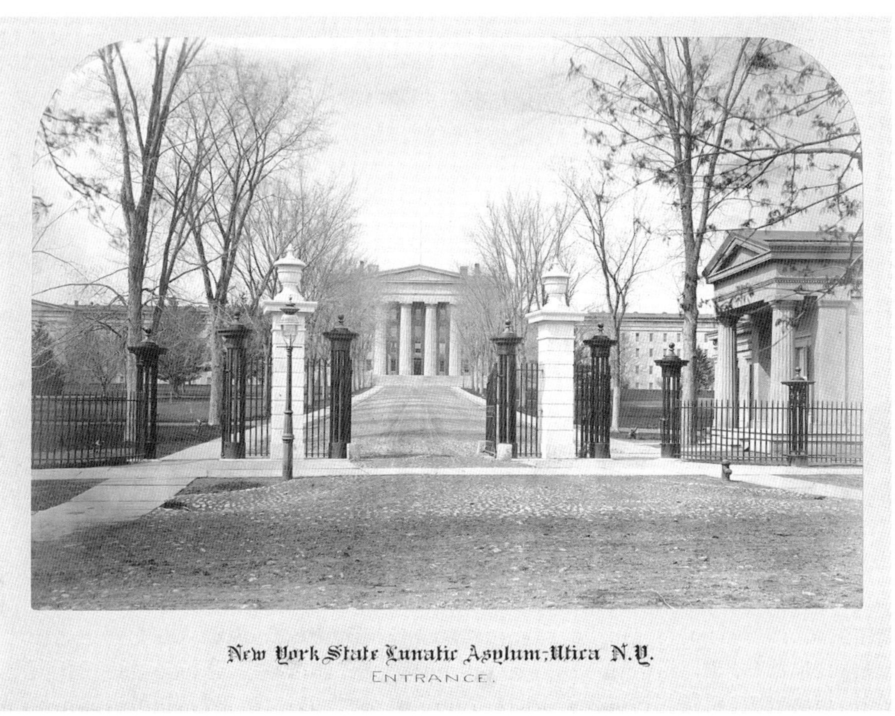

Patients would be escorted down this path to treatment. *New York State Archives.*

A Visit of the Legislature to the Lunatic Asylum

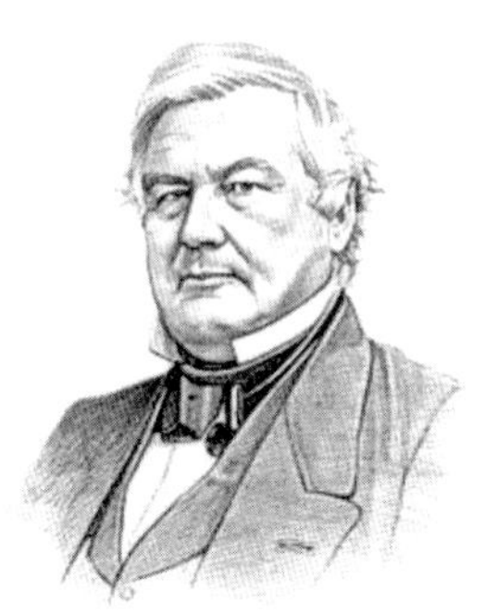

President Millard Fillmore (1850–1853) visited the Lunatic Asylum at Utica. *Oneida County History Center.*

On March 11, 1854, over one hundred New York State legislators and senators paid a visit to the Lunatic Asylum at Utica. This number also included many wives and staff. They had been invited by the administration of the asylum, for they were proud of the establishment as rumors of the innovative program spread across the country. In the past decade, the asylum had many visitors from other states, including the western territories of Illinois and Michigan. Many were administrators from other asylums who wanted to build a model like the one in Utica or see if the facility lived up to its illustrious reputation. These were a smattering of professionals, but the official visit by a large portion of the New York State legislature was cause for celebration.

After resting from their trip, the entire procession was escorted into the state parlor, where the culinary expertise of the patients was put on display. The state's political elite did not have a royal food taster, so they had to dive into the food and drink with nary a hesitation. The Honorable Joseph Benedict of Utica welcomed the group and then turned them over to a meal of roasted turkey, ham and "incomparable pickles." At the conclusion of dinner, different legislators stood up and addressed the crowd and particularly complimented the pickles. The group was then led on a tour of the asylum departments and took great joy in seeing the print shop. After the tour, the entire group went into the chapel, along with patients, and had a church service. The sermon was one of happiness and praise in New York State having abolished slavery, built the Erie Canal and then constructed the Lunatic Asylum at Utica. After many lengthy addresses, the group proceeded back to the dining hall to partake in ice cream and coffee. The patients were overjoyed to receive visitors, and the legislators seemed pleased with the state's investment. The legislatures then left the asylum, climbed into their carriages and traveled back to Albany.

The address to everyone in attendance was given by the Honorable Benjamin Joy, who spoke on behalf of the Senate and Assembly, which had

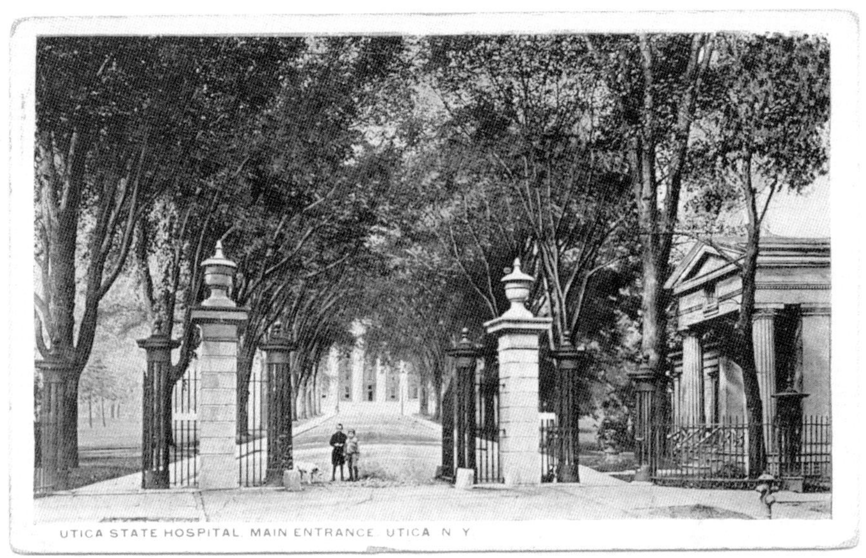

This postcard was sent to a family member from the newly named Utica State Hospital, as lunatic asylum was no longer appropriate. *Courtesy Dennis Webster.*

made building the asylum a reality. H.C. Paige printed Joy's remarks in the *Albany Register*. The following is taken word-for-word from this address:

> *That which has been witnessed to-day, is too touching, too deeply affecting to pass unnoticed, and yet, how can language express the feelings which well up in the heart, and give utterance in copious tears, as we look upon the inmates of this institution, and listen to their various utterances.*
>
> *I never felt such unmingled pride and admiration for my country, and her noble institutions, as I do at this hour. As members of the Legislature, there have been before us deaf and dumb. By our system of educating that class, the deaf are made, if not to hear, at least to understand, and the dumb to speak in a written language.*
>
> *The idiot, from the dark, deep mental chaos which enshrouded him, has, by our institutions for his instruction, been brought to a state of mental capacity and enjoyment. A change has been wrought in this once forsaken and hopelessly abandoned class, which staggers belief, and must be witnessed to be in any degree appreciated. We have seen those, who had once been regarded as hopelessly idiotic, who could not feed themselves, capable of observing and appreciating, and able to comprehend figures, and*

to understand many different branches of study. Indeed, such development of mind as lift them fairly above their former condition, and make them a comfort to their kindred and themselves.

And what is the spectacle presented here before us? We here learn, that this one noble institution, for the aid of that most unfortunate class, who find aid and comfort within these walls, has in its short period of its existence, aided over four thousand persons, and now has nearly four hundred and fifty in charge and under treatment.

How sincerely should we exult in these great systems of benevolence, which look after the wretched of our land. Are they not God like? Did not the Saviour of mankind make the miserable—the blind—the halt—the maimed—the deaf—the dumb—and the insane, his special care? In what shall we exalt so much then, as in those Heaven-born institutions, whose office it is to emulate his illustrious example?

Of the causes of insanity, this may not be the appropriate place for me to speak, but it is highly fitting for me to say, that if these causes are in whole, or in ever so small a degree, under human control, the highest Christian obligation demands not only a search for those causes, but their prompt removal. The eloquent speaker who preceded me has pointed you to one great cause- the liquor traffic. May this cause be speedily removed. Do we not feel today a deep impression that humanity demands it?

To the inmates of this institution let me say that you have our deepest sympathies. Our hearts go out toward you with gushing commiseration, and we involuntarily say, "how can we solace your sorrows?" We will remember you as legislators—we will remember you as your fellow-citizens, and liable to all your griefs. We will remember you in our families, when we each return to our homes, and our little ones gather around us to learn of what we have seen in our absence; we will speak to them of you- and when we offer the morning and evening acknowledgements to Heaven, then shall our prayers ascend to that God, who "as a father pitieth his children, so pitieth he them that fear him," that you may be in his holy keeping and be restored to health, and to your anxious friends.

Who, of all present, possessed of unclouded reason, will he be henceforth thankful for this inestimable gift? Who, but will be more deeply touched with sympathy for the suffering? Who, that is a father, but will cling more tenderly to his children, and bless the "giver of all good," that they are distinguished from the insane, and exempted from their sorrows? And who, but will feel increased concern, to shield his offspring from every cause, whether near or remote, which can produce the melancholy results which we have to-day witnessed?

What citizen of the Empire State, but will feel prouder of his State, and more determined to prove himself worthy of her high renown, and more zealously to foster her noble and God-like "State Charitable Institutions?" Not one, I feel assured, within whose bosom reigns a love of country, a generous heart, and a sympathetic pity for the unfortunate!

Two Years and Three Months in the N.Y. Lunatic Asylum at Utica

The picture of lunatic asylum life portrayed in the *Opal* puts a positive spin on the operations and running of the facility. Like everything in life, there are two sides to every story. Critics of the *Opal* have stated that it was filled with letters of former patients praising their care, optimistic stories and flowery poetry. Reading the entire span of the nine-year run, there is plenty of that, but there are some snippets of the life inside the Lunatic Asylum at Utica. In 1855, Phebe B. Davis published a paper titled "Two Years and Three Months in the N.Y. State Lunatic Asylum at Utica." It's a fascinating paper written right after her release from the asylum. Davis wrote of the issues she faced while in the asylum, including her witnessing what she described as abuse. Davis described herself as a sane and educated Yankee woman who was not a "crazy head" and did not belong in the asylum.

When she arrived, she was taken in to meet with Dr. Benedict, who was the supervising superintendent at that time. She described the doctor as "smooth as glass" and unemotional. She said he was "bland and a perfect specimen of amiability." She stated they sat her in a room with paper and pen and asked her many questions about her background and mental condition. She was exhausted at the end of this lengthy interview. Davis was admitted and taken to the fourth hall, where her bonnet and shawl were taken. She sat by the window and said the other female patients, twenty to thirty in number, of the hall came right up to her and stared like children. She called their faces vacant with disconnected conversations.

Davis feared for her life and did not sleep, as she felt she was surrounded by murderers. She claimed they tried to drive out her insanity by brute force. She stated the doctors strolled around in a cool, forbidding manner with cold indifference toward the patients. She referred to the staff as "ignorant Irish Catholics," "Welch dough-heads" and "Yankee greenhorns." She called the doctors "ignoramuses." Phebe Davis was an educated and bright woman who liked to tell the reader how savvy and smart she is. She called all the other female patients crazy and wondered why she had been committed to the asylum. She did acknowledge Dr. Benedict as a great man but then called him small and insignificant. She said that some of the ladies were quite intelligent and did not belong there but that there were a number who would need to be in the asylum forever. She did not like patients harnessed to their beds even though they had mania. She said that she had seen horses treated better. Davis claimed she would eat all her meals in the water closet of the asylum. Eventually, she was deemed cured and released. She wrote her memoirs from sheets of secret code she compiled while in Old Main. She claimed to do this because the superintendent would take her manuscript if he was able to read what she had written. It's a fascinating tale written by a woman in the midst of her being committed and treated.

Dorothea Dix

Dorothea Dix (1802–1887) was a most prominent advocate for the rights and humane treatment for those with mental illness. Her visit to the Lunatic Asylum at Utica resulted in a conversation between two patients. The interaction was reported in the January 1857 issue of the *Opal*. Dix was walking down the main hall of the asylum, passing by patients, when a younger girl called together some ladies and asked, "Who was that lady?" and one of the women present replied, "That was Miss Dix, the philanthropist." The girl scrunched her eyebrows and, with a blank expression, asked, "What is a philanthropist, please?" Another replied, "Philanthropist, my dear, is a word from two Greek words, signifying a lover of men." The girl nodded, smiled and said, "Well, then, are not all we women philanthropists?" Dorothea spent her life traveling across Europe and the United States advocating for the proper care of those with mental illness. She began her career as a schoolteacher and started to visit jails. On such visits, she noticed that those with mental illness were placed in jails alongside killers and was outraged at being told that lunatics had no feelings. She shared a philosophy with Dr.

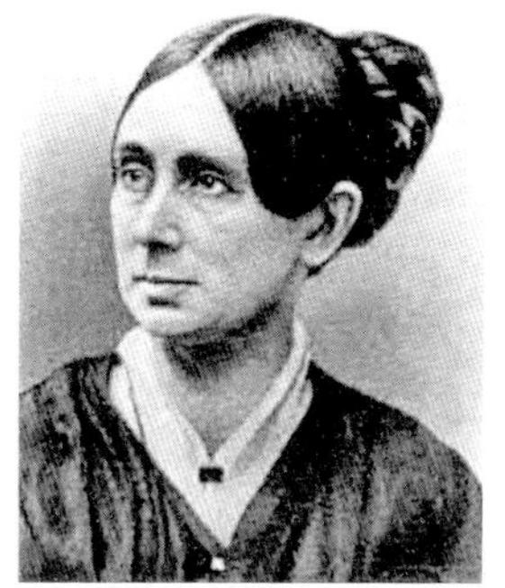

World-renowned mental health patient advocate Dorothea Dix. *Oneida County History Center.*

Brigham: those with mental illness could be cured and deserved to be treated with dignity and proper care. Today she is considered a pioneer in loving treatment to those with mental illness.

Gerrit Smith

The most famous patient of the asylum, Gerrit Smith, was a national leader in the abolition movement. There are many who viewed enslaved people's fight for freedom similar to the plight of those afflicted with mental disabilities. The "lunatics" of the mid-nineteenth century often had their own freedom ripped away and were placed into seclusion, sometimes for the rest of their lives. New York State declared slavery illegal in the 1850s, and Gerrit Smith was right in the middle of the movement to free the slaves. Based in Peterboro, New York, Smith was a highly regarded and well-respected abolitionist who financially assisted many, including John Brown. Smith was part of the "Secret Six," a group of six wealthy supporters who funded the antislavery efforts of John Brown, who had increasingly moved toward the creed of action more than of advocacy. The raid on the United States arsenal at Harper's Ferry, led by John Brown, was one of the contributing factors of the start of the Civil War. On October 16, 1859, Brown, his sons and followers failed to take the armory and were captured by locals and troops. After being found guilty of treason, John Brown was hanged. There was a check written by Gerrit Smith in Brown's pocket when he was captured. This led many to believe that Smith knew about the raid and had funded it. Senator Jefferson Davis attempted to have Smith tried and hanged for his involvement in the raid. Smith admitted himself into the Lunatic Asylum at Utica, claiming mental breakdown from the stress of the raid and the aftermath. Many thought that perhaps Smith faked his mental illness to keep from going on trial. It has never been proven that Smith knew about the raid, and he certainly would have received the best mental health treatment in the world during his stay at the asylum.

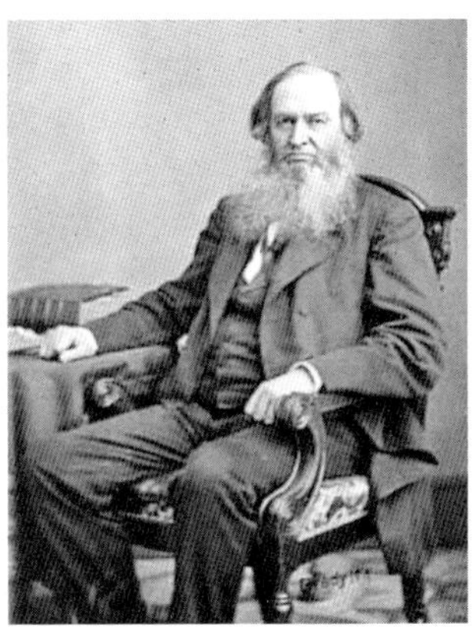

Abolitionist Gerrit Smith, who placed himself in the Lunatic Asylum at Utica. *Oneida County History Center.*

ANNUAL REPORT OF THE MANAGERS OF THE STATE LUNATIC ASYLUM (1869)

Since the opening of the asylum in 1843, an annual report was presented to the managers, who would present the findings to New York State. The main function was to keep the state legislature abreast of the goings-on at the asylum. The report of 1869 was the twenty-sixth; it was transmitted to the legislature in January, so the report covers the operating year of 1868.

Officers of the Asylum

MANAGERS
Christopher Morgan
Edmund Graham
Daniel P. Bissell, MD
Spencer Kellogg
Francis Kernan
Samuel Campbell
Hiram Denio
O.B. Matteson
S.O. Vanderpoel, MD

TREASURER
Edmund A. Wetmore

RESIDENT OFFICERS
John P. Gray, MD—Superintendent and Physician
A.O. Kellogg, MD—First Assistant Physician
Judson B. Andrews, MD—Second Assistant Physician
Walter Kempster, MD—Third Assistant Physician
Horatio N. Dryer—Steward
Emma Barker—Matron

SPECIAL PATHOLOGIST
E.R. Hun, MD

The opening letter of the report stated that at the end of the year 1868, there were 603 patients in the asylum and 985 treated that year; 58 patients died.

They had admitted since the 1843 opening 8,762 patients. Overcrowding was addressed but praise listed for the two new asylums being constructed in New York State. One interesting note was the water supply had been coming from lock number 5 of the Chenango Canal and was being pumped up to the asylum through iron pipes. These pipes froze during the winter, leaving the asylum without ample water. Snow and ice had to be melted to supply water. A steam engine was purchased to keep this from happening the following winter. They reported that 24 patients had come to the asylum in chains and some with their arms tied behind their backs with rope. All were unchained and untied before entering the asylum.

The report has details on everything from number admitted to number of meals each patient received during the year. The number of days spent in bed was also listed and broken down by month. The report stated that people kept showing up to see the patients then commenting that they were disappointed that they cannot see the most mad in their insane state. They wanted to see the worst patients, "the raving crazy ones." The managers felt that this practice had to stop, as these visitors could agitate and reverse months of treatment. They also believed it was best to separate the patients by sanity classifications. There has always been an urban legend surrounding Old Main that people were kept in chains in the basement. This is false, as even in the board of manager's report, they mentioned they had conducted their annual visit and inspection of the Lunatic Asylum at Utica and found "the entire absence of a dungeon and chains." The managers reported that the fiscal books looked sound, the asylum clean and the staff hard at work.

The educational levels of the patients offer an interesting statistic in the report: of 382 admissions to the asylum, only 7 had a college degree and only 27 could read and write. The majority were married men and women, with only 1 divorced man. Occupations listed included 103 housekeepers, 61 farmers, 34 laborers, 8 teachers, 4 lawyers and many other occupations. The top manias listed for those admitted were melancholia, acute mania and dementia. Inventory listed included almost 4,000 sheets, pillowcases, towels and other articles. The farm and garden had stock listed of apples, beans, celery, corn, hay and many other fruits and vegetables. The farm listed 8 horses, 1 pony, 2 oxen, 1 bull, 1 yearling, 3 calves, 31 cows and 110 hogs. Dr. Gray ended the report with a message of thanks to the board of managers and the legislature.

"TREATMENT OF THE INSANE IN NEW YORK STATE" (1879)

In an article in the November 23, 1879 issue of the *New York Herald*, Dr. William A. Hammond was interviewed and asked his opinion on the treatment of asylum patients in New York, as well as his view on the Utica crib restraining device. Dr. Hammond was an expert on diseases of the mind and spoke quite openly and honestly about the asylums. He stated that the physicians in charge were more concerned with financial matters of the asylum, running the farm and electioneering with members of the legislature than practicing proper medicine. He was especially harsh about the treatment of the patients and the use of the Utica crib. He said the nurses were brutal and ignorant and used the cribs without the orders or supervision of the doctors. Dr. Hammond added that nurses would inflict corporal punishment, beating, flogging, knocking down and stamping on patients. He said the force feeding of patients was terrible and that the commissioner who inspected the asylums was fooled—asylum staff knew of the visit and prepared to show their best behavior. Dr. Hammond stated that England's institutions were much advanced, as they had eliminated bars on windows and restraints on insane patients. He said the only time a patient should be restrained is during surgical procedures.

Dr. Hammond mentioned censoring patient letters was a grave injustice and that a single superintendent should be abolished and the asylums run like a hospital, with a team of physicians. He said lunatics were sick people, not possessed by the devil. A patient in an asylum should be safe and protected.

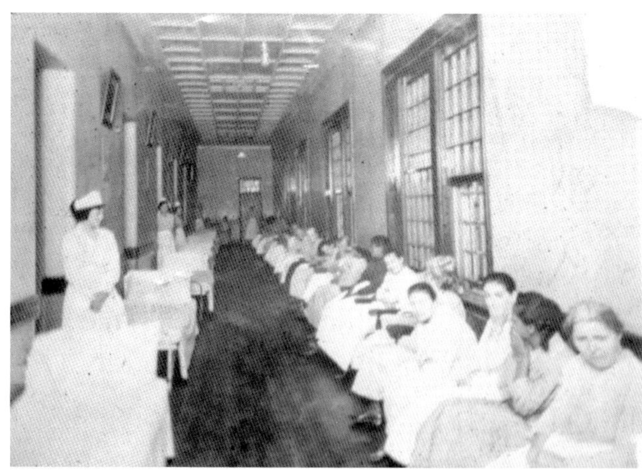

Halls became crowded as patient numbers swelled. *New York State Archives.*

The doctor stated that the system of employment in asylums needed to improve. The one in Utica had some good employment, but others had nothing at all, which made patients sit all day with nothing to do.

Dr. Hammond's harshest words were for the Utica crib, the restraining device invented in Utica by Dr. Brigham. It was still used not only in New York State but also in asylums nationwide. He called the crib a coffin with barely enough room to move and asserted that patients died in the device. It was an unscientific, barbarous instrument. He felt insanity was intensified in patients locked horizontally inside, as the blood flowed improperly inside the brain. He thought a padded room was a much better alternative to the Utica crib. The doctor concluded that the aura of mystery surrounding asylums must disappear. Acts of tyranny and oppression by the attendants must be stopped. Asylums should be upgraded with new leaders who came from the field of studying the mind who could use their advanced knowledge to improve treatment and conditions of those suffering with mental illness.

An Inner View of the State Lunatic Asylum at Utica (1881)

This book was published by attorney William L. Trull after he was committed for insanity. It's a fascinating and rare view of the inside workings of the asylum. In his introduction, Trull stated, "The object of this little book is to create a feeling of public sympathy for the insane which shall result in a correction of the abuses of which it complains. With this in view I call upon the friends of humanity everywhere to aid in its circulation." This author is sure Trull would be pleased that his words are still being read long after his demise. There's an interesting note that he entered the work into Congress in 1881 as a matter of permanent public record. Trull said that his mental condition began in 1877, when he had become mentally and physically feeble in his hometown of Cohoes, New York. He felt better and opened his law office in January 1878, but after a few months of practicing law, he fell ill again and had to abandon his business. His insanity he described as "melancholia." He said mental illness is the worst disease known to man.

Trull felt himself slipping into the maelstrom of madness, and in fighting the king of terrors, he lacked sleep and had trouble eating. He'd lie awake all night long. It was at this time that he had suicidal thoughts. He traveled to the city in order to kill himself. He went to Dr. T (he didn't give the full name) and was given a shot in his arm of morphia and a prescription for a bottle of hydrate of chloral. Trull purchased some writing materials. He went to a hotel, penned his suicide note to family and friends and gave the message to a hotel porter. Trull went back into his room and stood in the window looking over the city and guzzled the entire bottle of the prescribed medicine. He passed out in his bed and was saddened to awaken to relatives and doctors by his bedside. They had saved him, and he was sent to the asylum at Taunton, Massachusetts. While there, Trull was able to get a piece of broken glass from a window and slashed his arm. A quick move by an attendant saved his life, and he was outfitted in a straitjacket for the remainder of his time at the asylum. Trull tried to bribe his six roommates to loosen his straitjacket, but they would not. The night watchman would come in the room with a lantern and look at him in the face to see if he was still alive. Trull would be released after seventeen days at Taunton.

Trull next wrote about paying a visit to the Utica Asylum. He wanted to see what he called the "model institution" known worldwide. He called Dr. John P. Gray a genius in his supervision but mainly from his writings and publication of the *American Journal of Insanity* at the Utica facility. Trull had read the Annual Report of the Managers from 1878, which invited the public to come to the asylum and see it for themselves. He quoted the report directly:

> *The asylum has continued open to public visitation as for a number of years past. I am well satisfied that free admission of visitors has no injurious influence upon the patients, but on the contrary is productive of good. For a number of years we have employed Mr. George Millham, an intelligent and judicious man, who attends to the duty of showing visitors through the wards. The institution is thus seen in its general arrangements and workings at all times. Though the general regulation for visiting is from two to five in the afternoon, there are so many persons from out of the city, who come during the morning hours, that we are obliged to make very large exceptions to the rule. While information is freely given touching the general arrangements, all proper privacy is preserved in regard to the names, personal history, and conduct of the patients. The number of patients during the year was 7,825. Besides this, the number of persons who brought patients to the asylum also visited the wards of the institution. The record-book of visitation shows 1,988 visited their friends in the various wards of the asylum. All these, with the visitation by superintendents of the poor, and other public officers, make a list of more than 10,000.*

Trull stated that a few thousand of the annual visitors go to the Utica Asylum to satisfy themselves of the falsity of truth regarding the ill treatment of the unfortunate inmates. He wrote of getting off at the train station and taking a fifteen-minute ride by horse and buggy to the asylum. The first thing he saw was the magnificent front lawn of fourteen acres, which contrasted sharply with the massive granite prison with its "Bastille-like appearance." He mentioned forty to fifty patients out in the yard with attendants watching them, keeping them from jumping the fence and escaping. Attendants were allegedly docked five dollars in pay if a patient under their watch escaped, and it seems there were numerous attempts. Some of the patients were playing croquet or other games, and some were just standing there brooding. Trull heard an attendant telling patients the doctor ordered him to keep patients one hundred feet away from the fence lest they jump it and escape.

An attendant spoke to Trull about a gray-haired inmate who had been at the asylum for twenty-eight years, a veteran of the Mexican War, and was very happy. The attendant then pointed out a man with a neckerchief tied around his neck, as if covering a sore throat, but the man had recently attempted suicide and was referred to as a "morphine eater." The asylum employee pointed to an old man who he claimed had been there since the institution opened and had been tied to a tree while it was being finished. The man's insanity had occurred when he was a young man and was thrown from a horse and received a brain injury. The attendant took Trull over to the old man to say hello. The old man stated that his son was to marry Queen Victoria's daughter Beatrice and that he was worth eight hundred thousand million dollars and he was gifting his son fifty million as a marriage gift. There was a man sitting and pretending to cast a fishing line over the grass. Trull then heard a whistle, and all the patients walked back inside the asylum. As they were walking up the stone steps, Trull heard one of the patients say, "open sesame." Trull and the other visitors were taken to a room by a polite little office boy to await the usher. He referred to the guide as fifty years old and with a pleasant face and disposition.

The tour began with a door being unlocked; then the group and the guide stepped inside and were locked in the asylum. The two-hundred-by-eighteen-foot hall was neat, clean and had a home-like appearance. Trull mentioned the decorations on the wall, including a framed motto, "With malice to none and charity to all." He went down the hall and saw twenty-five patients who did not seem to have the mannerisms of the insane. He noted some playing chess and checkers and one man on the piano. He heard a group of several men in a room laughing and chatting and thought to himself, "Can this be an insane asylum?" Trull took it as more of a first-class hotel. He wondered if the tour was staged to only show the best wards. They were brought through the chapel and the amusement room, where plays were staged and bands performed. He felt the tour soft-soaped the asylum and made it appear a wonderful home for the living dead.

William Trull returned home, yet only a few months later, his mania returned. On December 7, 1878, he was placed in the New York State Lunatic Asylum at Utica. He spent fourteen months at the Utica asylum and used his stay as the basis for his book. When he arrived, he was grilled with questions by a doctor who was determining his level of insanity and in which of the twelve rooms he would be placed. After this, Trull was deemed a number 7, which meant he was placed in room 7 of the men's wing. He learned that number 7 was called the "stuffing room" because the majority of the twenty patients inside refused to eat and had to be stuffed or force fed. Trull heard one doctor giving orders to a staff member, while pointing to a man who would not eat, "Stuff this man and make him fat." Trull described the man in charge of watching over 7 as large and powerful. He said the room was dimly lit and was around one hundred by fourteen feet. His bed was the most uncomfortable he had ever slept on, and his roommates were loud, disruptive, moaned all night and created a "perfect pandemonium." He described one man as praying aloud all night long and cursing all day long and another who would repeat and chant the same phrase over and over and over again. On top of all that, the night watchman came through once an hour with his lantern, coughing and waking everyone up in the room. Trull claimed he did not sleep at all his first six nights at the asylum.

Trull witnessed people being held in the Utica crib and called the device "abominable" and "an instrument of torture." He felt only the most insane should even be considered to be placed in this device. He felt the narrow cage with the locking lid would aggravate and disturb rather than calm and cure. He could not imagine the suffering of those locked in it for ten-hour stretches at night. He claimed that he saw the device being used on at least three wards and the attendants used it to punish the patients for minor infractions. He related the tale of a patient named Brown who, when it was bedtime, pleaded with the attendant not to place him back in the crib. He was afraid he would be caught in the device and perish if a fire were to hit the asylum. The attendant told Brown to stop being a nuisance and get in the crib. He said if Brown rattled the cage like he had the night before, he would be removed and dunked in a cold bath. When Brown tried to debate with the attendant, Trull claimed that the staff member and a few others beat Brown with repeated blows until he undressed and climbed into the Utica crib. After he was locked in the crib, the attendant said, "Good night, Mr. Brown." Trull was thankful he was never placed in the Utica crib and called it a barbarous device. He mentioned seeing straitjackets, wrist restraints and waist restraints while at the asylum.

The muff is a restraining device Trull described as going up to the elbows, covering the hands and forearms of the patient, who is then strapped to a chair sitting up. This allowed the attendant to "stuff" the face of the patient with food if they had refused to eat. He said a patient named Jones had refused to open his mouth to eat when the attendant punched him in the stomach to get him to open his mouth. If this didn't work, they would choke a patient and always did so in full view of the other patients. What Trull called "gruel" was nothing more than bread mixed in with milk that would be force-fed to patients. When the stuffing process did not work, Trull described the next step as "tubing." They would insert a metal device in the mouth, cranked open with a thumbscrew to hold the mouth open. The patient was tied down with the muff so they could not fend off this process. Then a rubber tube would be snaked down the throat into the stomach. A funnel was attached to the tube, and then life-sustaining fluids were poured down the tube until the man was full. They would repeat this on the other patients who refused to eat.

Trull talked about how four times a day a cart would come around with their medicinal treatments and the attendant would say, "Medicine, gentlemen." This made Trull laugh, as he said they'd be called gentlemen yet thumped in the ribs if they refused to take their medicine. Trull noted that the men who refused their medicine would be forced to take it by three large attendants. One would hold the arms down, one would choke the man by the throat and the third would pour the medicine down. Trull said they cooperated, but some would hold the medicine in their throat, then at the first chance spit it out the window. One patient described the asylum as "Utica Hell." The men in 7 quickly realized Trull was an educated man who could read and write letters and asked for his assistance. He mentioned one patient who thought snakes were slithering over his body and prayed day and night for them to go away. This patient would bash his own ears to get rid of them, and they became bloody and misshapen. Trull described patients being battered, pummeled and abused for not following the orders of the attendants and lamented that such things were allowed.

Trull said the asylum was not living up to its reputation, and the most abused patient he witnessed while committed was a male patient in 7 whom he called J.K. Trull described the man as a living skeleton and worthy of a part in a Barnum attraction. This man was the most wretched and feeble human he had ever witnessed. J.K. was pummeled numerous times and force-fed for refusing to eat his food. The patients lacked the courage and the strength to report these abuses to the doctors. Trull was moved to ward number 2, thus leaving behind his friends. He did sleep better, as the patients were quieter in that ward. Trull started to write down the abuses he saw and was mocked, he said, by assistant physicians who said nobody would ever believe him. After months in this hall, Trull was promoted to ward number 1, where the highest functioning and least insane patients were kept. Trull said in his time there, men in ward number 3 had the greatest number of releases and only surmised as that's where the farmers were kept together. Trull mentioned that the bars on the windows in ward 1 were there to keep burglars out but not to keep the patients from escaping. One huge benefit was he could now shave himself instead of an attendant doing it, armed with a dull razor. He was also allowed to sit in the front row on Sunday church services. Trull said that the attendants were of a higher quality in the lower numbered wards and spoke much nicer to the patients, so much so that he said it was patronizing. He said it was better than being in what was referred to as the "black eye" wards.

The narrative mentioned a couple suicide attempts, including one where the man cut his throat and his tongue with a razor. The man recovered, but his speech was impaired from his mangled tongue. Of the attempts mentioned, only three were successful. Trull enjoyed being put to work, using a hand lawn mower to cut the asylum grass. He liked the work and the fresh air and became a model patient, increasingly given freedom and duties such as being the knife counter. He gathered and counted the knives after every meal, as patients had to return them after they ate. Trull mentioned being able to go to the grand ballroom for a celebration of a returning doctor, and the lovely music drowned out the wails and moans of the patients. It was the first time in his stay that he heard something else. For some reason not listed, Trull was then moved to ward 6. A fellow patient named Pat died of starvation, as the man could not keep anything down, claiming he had an ill-tempered stomach. It bothered Trull that Pat refused to lie in a bed as he died, as he didn't want to upset the attendants—they greatly disliked anybody messing up their beds during the day. It upset Trull that this man died sitting up in a chair and not in the comfort of a bed with a soft pillow. Trull did say the food was plentiful, good and offered choice; although not the tastiest, it was sufficient. He said the theory at Utica was that if a man was fat, he was sane.

Trull found ward 6 not as good as 1 and was annoyed at the attendant who would not allow the patients sufficient time to eat their meals. Less than five minutes to eat and wash their dishes was the norm. Trull mentioned a patient in 6 named Billings who was outspoken. He had been injured when a patient was thrown down the stairs by an angry attendant and landed on him. When Billings complained, the attendants rained blows down on him. They removed Billings to ward 8, and the next time Trull saw him, the man had a sling on his arm. Trull then described a small man with a black eye approaching the touring doctor on the ward. The man said he was praying to Moses in the Utica crib and the attendants were so angry they took him out of it and punched him until he stopped praying. "How can you deny this?" asked the patient as he pointed to his black eye. "You call this a lunatic asylum? I say it is a devilish pounding factory." Trull stated that this unnamed doctor chuckled and walked away. The most dangerous part was the attendants calling out the man for telling the doctor.

Fear kept most from reporting anything, as the doctors would leave and the patients were alone with their abusers. Trull did say some of the doctors were tenderhearted, so he wondered why they would not discharge these thugs. Many were cured and released, but the abuse he witnessed was on four different wards with the patients deemed incurable. And in his opinion, this kind of treatment was not only at Utica but also all facilities for the insane in the United States. Dr. Gray, the superintendent of the asylum when Trull was there, said to him, "Mr. Trull you are forever troubling yourself about the misfortunes of others instead of looking out for yourself." Trull had started to write everything down that he witnessed in a diary. Trull asserted that he was not afraid to dress down attendants and speak his mind about the things he witnessed. He was not "clay to the hands of the potter." Trull did say there were many warm and friendly attendants whom he admired at the asylum. Trull was able to openly communicate with friends by penning letters and handing them to boys through the fence to mail for him. He said the asylum administration opened all letters and didn't allow any to leave that had anything bad to say about their care. Trull did let Dr. Gray know he was going to publish his book on the asylum treatment once he got out.

After he was released, Trull wrote that after Dr. Gray was criticized for using the Utica crib, he had a reporter from a newspaper climb inside in order to prove a man could move while locked inside. Trull wrote his book from memory, as he claimed that all his letters, notes and diaries were taken by the attendants and never returned. He called the Utica Asylum a "hellish paraphernalia of torture." Trull's wife eventually arrived at the asylum and asked that her husband be released. Dr. Gray obliged, and Trull was discharged. He concluded that the practices he witnessed, as well as the Utica crib, should be "consigned to the oblivion of the past."

Part II

Utica State Hospital (1890–1973)

G. Alder Blumer, MD (1886–1899)

Dr. G. Alder Blumer was appointed superintendent on December 19, 1886, replacing the long-tenured and much beloved Dr. Gray. Dr. Blumer was interested in modern advancements to assist those suffering mental illness and had started at the asylum as a fourth assistant physician but quickly rose to second in command. He took a trip to Europe to visit mental hospitals and witness their treatments, advancements he could bring back to Utica. Dr. Blumer would not waste time making changes. He started with opening a larger assembly hall on January 4, 1887, that would host weekly dances for the asylum patients. Activities increased under Dr. Blumer with the installation of organized sports for the patients, including a baseball team that played with great joy on the asylum grounds in August 1888. An athletic field day was held on August 29, 1887, and became an annual event thereafter. A Christmas tree party was held with staff and patients singing Christmas carols. This event proved popular. In 1888, the asylum purchased a boat called the *General Herkimer* and used it to take patients on rides on the Erie Canal. This was a very popular outing for the patients.

Dr. Blumer made two modern and drastic moves during his tenure. The Utica crib usage ended under Dr. Blumer when he had the last device removed from Utica State Hospital on January 18, 1887. The device that was born at the asylum had finally been banished. At the time, the press had referred to the device as an instrument of torture. Dr. Blumer was a student of Dr. Brigham's moral treatment and non-restraint patient care.

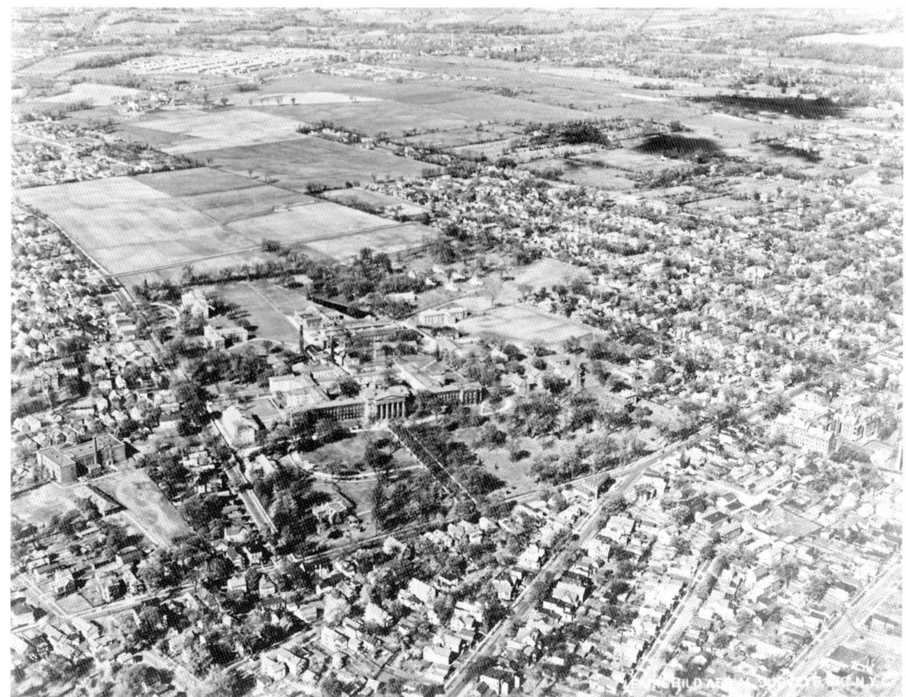

Overhead view of Utica State Hospital. *New York State Archives.*

Dr. Blumer's next move was to change the name from the Lunatic Asylum to Utica State Hospital. He had petitioned the New York State legislature to stop using the words *lunatic* and *asylum*. The legislature enthusiastically agreed and changed the name in 1890.

The building now had carpeting, curtains and nurses and attendants in fine uniforms. The nurses wore white outfits with white caps adorned with a blue stripe, and the men wore blue woolen sack suits with brass buttons that had the arms of New York State on them.

Dr. Blumer put an end to Utica State Hospital and the Old Main building being used as a tourist destination. In the beginning, gawkers were embraced because it was important to the legislature to show the New York State taxpayers that the significant amount of money used to build Old Main had been put to good use. The problem was the superintendents going back to Dr. Brigham all loathed this policy and felt the patients should not be on exhibition, especially when many visitors would request to see the worst patients and especially those confined to the Utica cribs. In 1889, Dr. Blumer changed it so only relatives and friends of patients could come inside unless it was a prearranged visit by a board member, a visiting physician or another person mandated to visit. The general public would no longer walk the halls of Utica State Hospital. Old Main continued to admit many, with 3,441 admitted in 1889.

Dr. Blumer had another innovation; he integrated care by placing female nurses in the male patient wards. No longer would men take care of only men and women take care of women. A big step forward in operations occurred under Dr. Blumer when $23,000 for an electric was approved for a plant that would provide updated lighting. The conversion contract was given to Edison General Manufacturing Company; the installation and use of electricity started in April 1888.

Dr. Blumer would see advancements in oversight with the expansion and creation of the New York State Commission for Lunacy. The three-person board would be required to visit every institution for the insane and patient care in New York State twice a year. The trio would report directly to the governor. In 1890, the State Care Act was passed. Dr. Blumer had contributed significantly to its writing and passage. The main item was breaking the state up into hospital territories, thus ending separate mental health patient care based on diagnosis. This meant that places like Willard no longer had patients with the highest levels of mania. Two types of hospitals would no longer be needed, and those who were paupers and in almshouses were now to be admitted and taken care of in the state mental hospitals.

Dr. Blumer made an important first at Utica State Hospital in 1891 when he appointed Dr. Clara Smith as the first woman physician at Old Main. By this time, the daily average of patients was at 786, with 1,171 having been treated that year. With the passage of the State Care Act, overcrowding had again happened at Old Main. Since the building was now undergoing constant repairs, outbuildings would be constructed, marking the first time that patients would get mental health care in Utica outside the hallowed walls of Old Main. Ground was broken on two infirmary or hospital buildings on August 4, 1891. These buildings would house 170 men and 90 women. The first infirmary opened in 1892 and in 1922 was named Walcott House in memory of W. Stuart Walcott, president of the board, upon his death. The second building housed employees. This residence could house twenty employees and keep them close to Old Main. The training school continued to expand and excel under the tutelage of Dr. Blumer. The number of certified nurses was 59 in 1892, which was the first year diplomas were awarded. The pupils had to pass oral and written exams. Pupils were not given an official graduation until 1909.

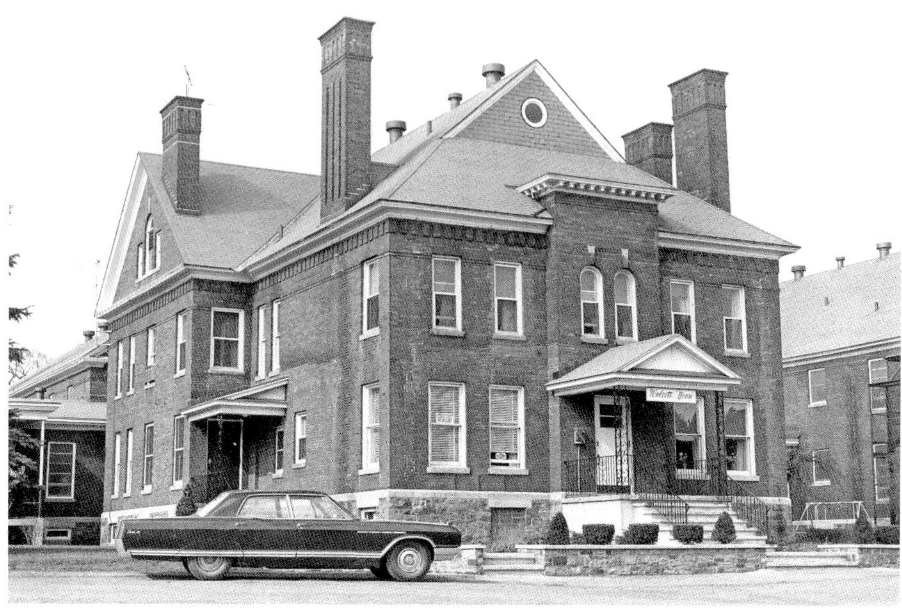

Walcott House on the Old Main campus. Opened in 1892, it was the infirmary at one time and hosted employees who were mandated to live on the campus. *New York State Archives.*

The biggest and most exciting advancement that happened under Dr. Blumer was the installation of what was referred to as a "rain bath." We call it a shower today, but on August 31, 1894, the rain bath was installed and began operating. Once again Old Main was at the forefront of innovation, as the first rain bath in New York State facilities was at the Utica State Hospital. In 1895, entrance exams were given to those wanting to get into the training school, which offered higher wages and two weeks of vacation. Dr. Blumer used these benefits to recruit and retain highly qualified employees.

Dr. Blumer expanded the farmland next to the asylum by leasing 160 acres south of the property; the expansion housed twenty male patients and was named Graycroft. The land would be purchased in 1900. A similar farmland purchase that employed twenty women patients was named Dixhurst. The ladies' property proved not as fruitful and was abandoned in 1901. These properties added 178 acres to the footprint of Utica State Hospital at a cost of around $35,000. The last innovative improvement under Dr. Blumer was in 1898, when a new water heater system was installed. Dr. Blumer resigned as superintendent of Utica State Hospital on September 4, 1899.

12TH Report of the New York Civil Service Commission (1895)

This report has the complete list of staff at Utica State Hospital, their positions and their salaries for the year 1895. The list includes those who were below the level of the physicians. There are 176 civil servant employees with 3 supervisors, 62 nurses, 56 attendants and a bunch of single occupations from baker and cook to soap maker and shoemaker. The top supervisor made $600 a year, nurses $144, attendants $312 and firemen $600.

Harold A. Palmer, MD (1899–1919)

Dr. Palmer would usher Old Main into the twentieth century when he replaced Dr. Blumer as the superintendent of Utica State Hospital. Dr. Palmer advocated a less stressful workplace for employees and implemented rotating staff for the most difficult patients. The practice of transporting employees into the city of Utica for ocular and dental services ended when they started bringing doctors into Old Main to keep patient care in-house. The number of patients coming in with geriatric issues like senility increased, and there was a syphilis outbreak. Dr. Palmer felt a separate home should be built for elderly patients, as they did not belong in a hospital for the mentally ill, but they had nowhere else to go. Dr. Palmer also lobbied and had built a separate building from Old Main that would house patients with communicable and infectious diseases. This isolation hospital opened in 1905 and admitted patients who were afflicted with tuberculosis, diphtheria and other diseases. The number of patients admitted in 1902 hit a high of 1,125.

Dr. Palmer continued Dr. Brigham's vision of moral treatment and had the occupational shops expanded. The patients started to manufacture clothing and other goods for other patients at hospitals across the state. A reception building was erected near Old Main, where those more acutely ill could be treated, and the facility, called Dunham Hall, opened in 1909. Utica was expanding, and people's homes started to encroach on the edge of the Old Main property. Noyes Street was the first right of way paved next to Utica State Hospital. The original name was Hickory Street. The Court Street cobblestone was replaced by modern pavement. The 1,400-foot frontage of Old Main received a nice flagstone sidewalk.

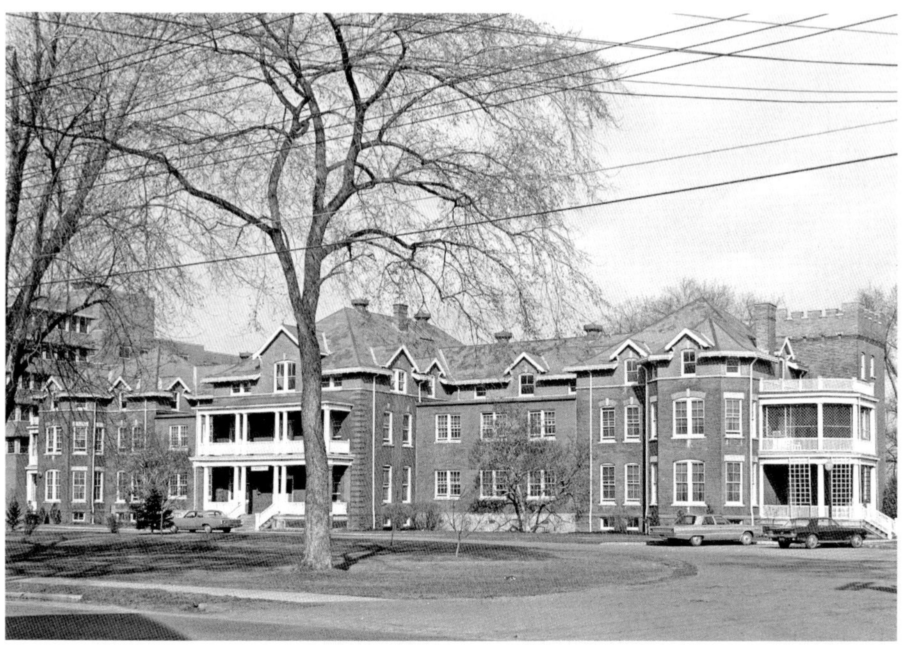

Dunham Hall on the Old Main campus. It opened in 1909 and was used for patient admittance before becoming a center for recreation programs. *New York State Archives.*

Dr. Palmer advanced the nursing school by hiring and appointing a woman to lead. Bessie B. Tibbettes, RN, became the nursing school superintendent as well as the instructor. A new laundry room was constructed, and admittance through Dunham Hall was implemented. Dr. Palmer increased outdoor activities for the patients and in 1913 started a reeducation school when he hired a young woman from the New Haven Normal School as the teacher. Dr. Palmer was a man married to his work and stayed a bachelor while the superintendent at Utica State Hospital. After twenty years of dedicated service as the superintendent, Dr. Palmer resigned due to health reasons.

RICHARD H. HUTCHINGS, MD (1919–1939)

Dr. Hutchings became the superintendent of Utica State Hospital on April 1, 1919, and ushered in an era of scientific advancement, increased community service and improved administrative efficiency. Dr. Hutchings was a different kind of man from all the previous superintendents, as he

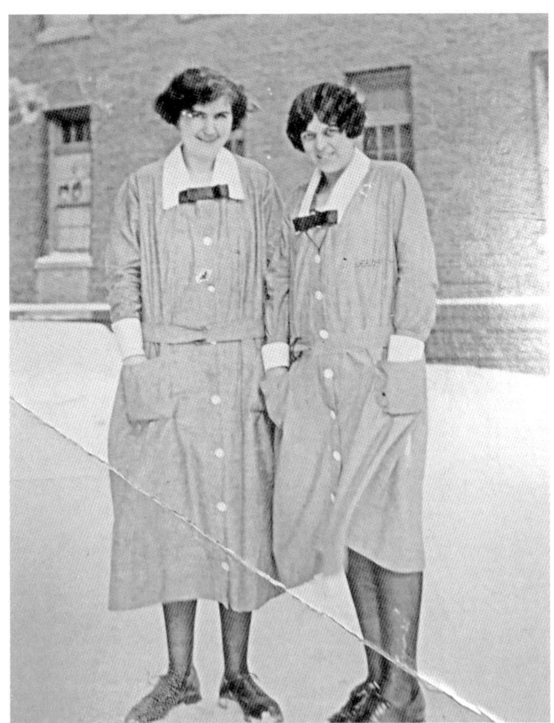

Left: Staff members outside. *New York State Archives.*

Below: Medicinal therapy advanced patient care. *New York State Archives.*

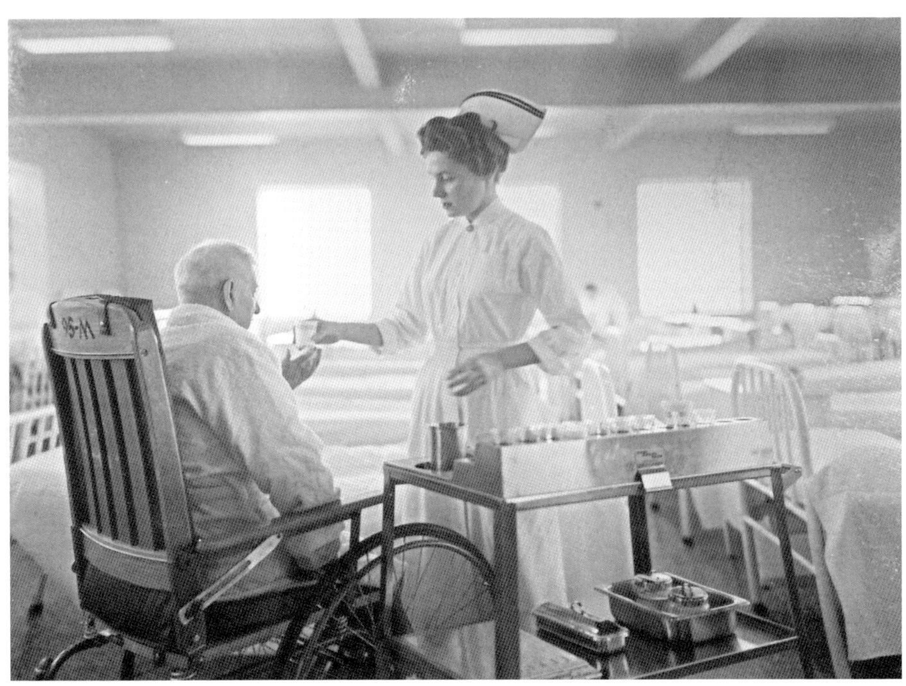

had vast private administrative experience and a military background. It would be these traits that endeared him to the board of managers and made for improvements in the administrative side of Utica State Hospital. Dr. Hutchings was a major in the U.S. Army Medical Corps, where he was chief of psychiatry and neurology. He served as the superintendent at the St. Lawrence State Hospital at the age of thirty-four. He was born in Clinton, Georgia and educated at Georgia Military School, Georgia University and New York's Bellevue Medical College. He came to Utica State a well-seasoned, worldly man.

Dr. Hutchings came on board when New York State purchased land in Marcy, New York, with the intentions of building a psychiatric center outside of the city of Utica. This structure was built under the guidance of Dr. Hutchings, and the first patients went to the Marcy facility in January 1923. He appointed Dr. Clarence O. Cheney as assistant superintendent and put him in charge of that building. By 1930, the Marcy building had more patients than Old Main. With over three thousand patients being ministered to annually, Dr. Hutchings recommended to the state that the Marcy facility be operated under its own superintendent. Dr. W.W. Wright became the first superintendent at the Marcy operation.

Dr. Hutchings oversaw major construction projects that improved Old Main and added more support for the hospital. Buildings were added that held the nurses' dining hall and apothecary clinic. The wards were

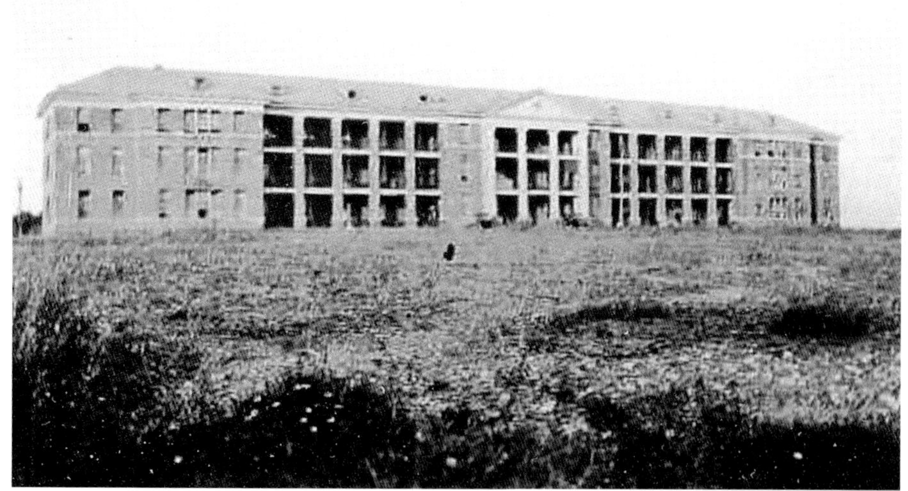

Marcy State Hospital opened in 1923 with patients transferred from Old Main. *Oneida County History Center.*

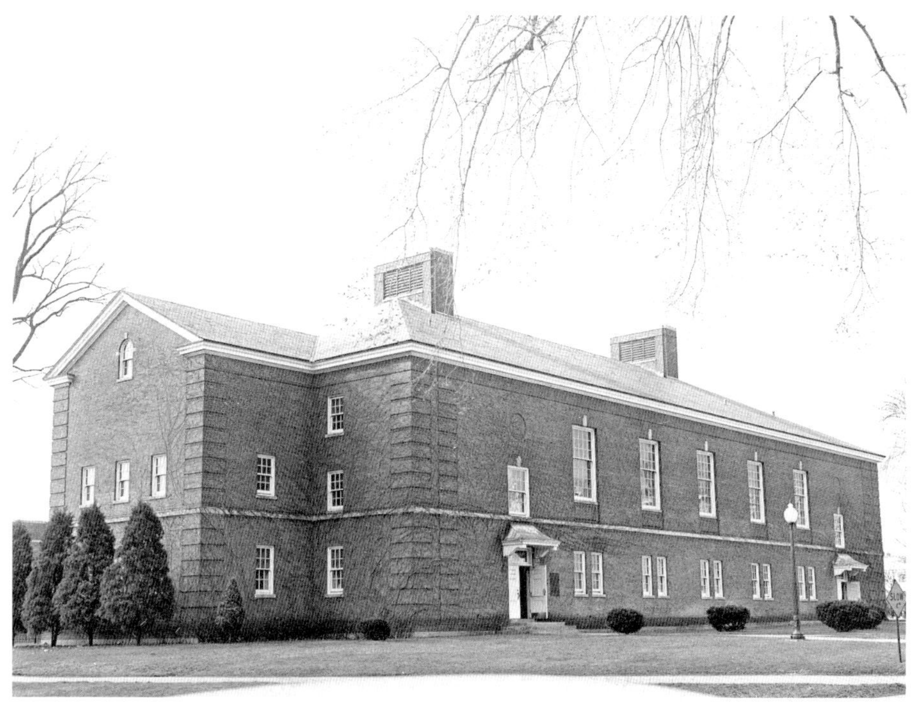

Hutchings Hall on the Old Main campus. Opened in 1938, this was where the business office was located. It also had an auditorium used for activities. *New York State Archives.*

remodeled and six cottages built for staff physicians. In 1925, the modern home for nurses was opened and named Dixhurst. The auditorium was the largest construction project and cost $300,000; it hosted church services, entertainment, scientific meetings and seminars. The structure would also host Utica public events. The new auditorium opened on October 5, 1938, and would be named Hutchings Hall after the beloved superintendent.

A new manufacturing facility was built that hosted a print shop and a coffee roasting facility. The coffee was stored, roasted and delivered to civil state hospitals throughout New York State. Many kinds of psychiatric publications, such as the *Psychiatric Quarterly*, the *Psychiatric Quarterly Supplement* and *Mental Hygiene News*, were printed in the building..

Utica continued to be a training ground for superintendents, with many starting their careers at Old Main before leaving Utica State Hospital for mental health facilities throughout New York. So many came from Old Main and ended up as superintendents nationwide that Utica State Hospital became known as the "mother of all hospitals." This moniker made Dr. Hutchings proud. Another advancement at Utica State Hospital was

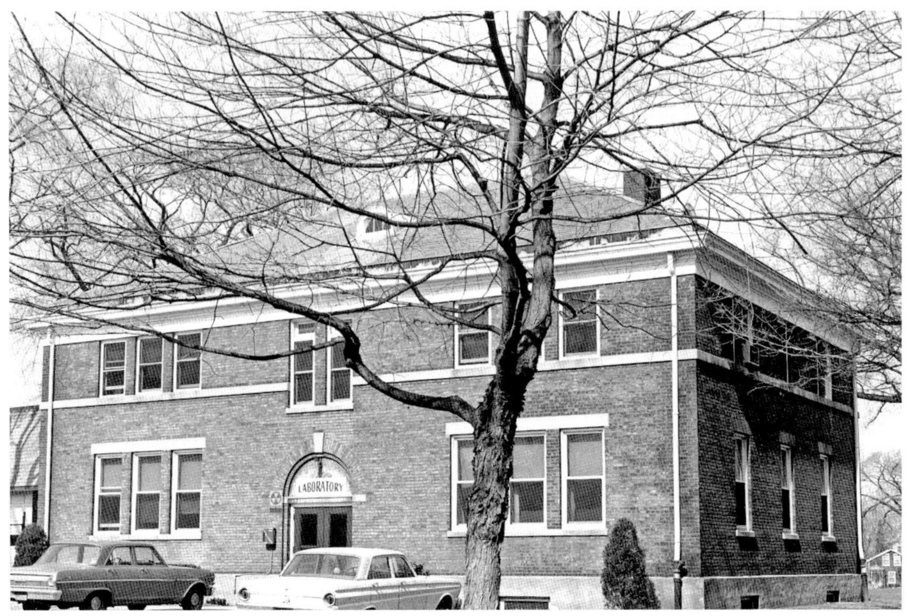

The laboratory on the Old Main campus, opened in 1920. Note the fallout shelter sign affixed to the building. *New York State Archives.*

expanding the education from superintendents and nurses to social workers. In the wake of the Great War, psychosocial services became popular. The laboratory was also used for educational and training purposes. Many college students flocked to Old Main to learn to serve those with mental illness. The social services department expanded when Dr. Hutchings appointed Eva M. Schied as director of social services and chief social worker.

Dr. Hutchings ended a long and stellar career at Utica State Hospital when, after twenty years, he retired on July 1, 1939. He was so esteemed that Syracuse employed him as a lecturer in psychiatry in its medical school and had an undergraduate medical society named after him. Dr. Hutchings wrote the *Psychiatric Word Book*, a popular text in most nursing schools.

Out of the Shadows Silent Film

Dr. Hutchings was advanced in many areas of study, including the medium of silent moving pictures. He oversaw the filming and production of a twenty-minute black-and-white silent film released about 1920 with the title

Out of the Shadows. It's about a fictional patient named Mary Hayes. Watching the movie is an educational experience, a snapshot in time. The film shows Mary's progress from diagnosis, admittance to the asylum, treatment, then dismissal.

The movie opens with the title: *Out of the Shadows*. The film looks very dark and grainy. The next words on the screen are a quote from Shakespeare: "Cans't thou not minister to a mind discard/Pluck from the memory a rooted sorrow/Raze out the written troubles of the brain/ Elas, with some sweet oblivious antidote/ Cleanse the foul bosom of that perilous stuff/Which weighs upon the heart."

The next title pops up: "Sometimes misfortune treads upon the heads of misfortune until the whole structure of life seems to crumble. The mind may give way under prolonged ill health and anxiety and the spectre MELANCHOLIA intrude when happiness should crown a long awaited day."

We then see a Model A car pull up to a house in Utica and a title reads, "The Doctor Arrives." The doctor comes out and goes into the house, where a sad-looking woman is holding a baby. They take her newborn, and the doctor looks her over. It looks like it's postpartum depression. Her head is down and shoulders slumped. The next title on screen says, "She is not improving. She cannot get well at home. She needs the care that can be given only in a mental hospital. I beg of you not to delay." We next see an asylum car arriving at the home and taking her away. The husband stands on the front porch holding the baby. The car arrives at Utica State Hospital building, and two nurses escort her into Dunham Hall. The title on screen says, "Receiving Ward." The

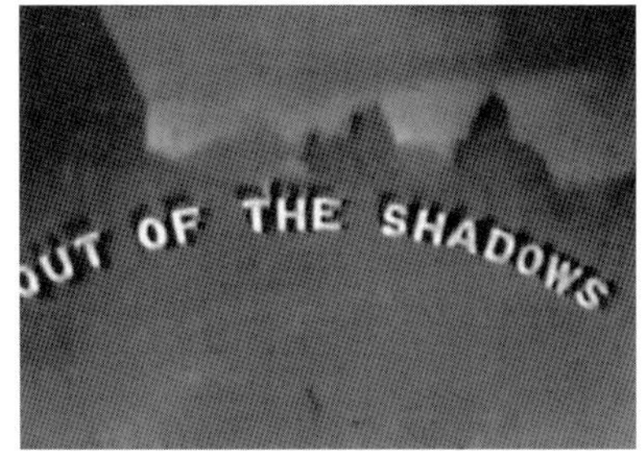

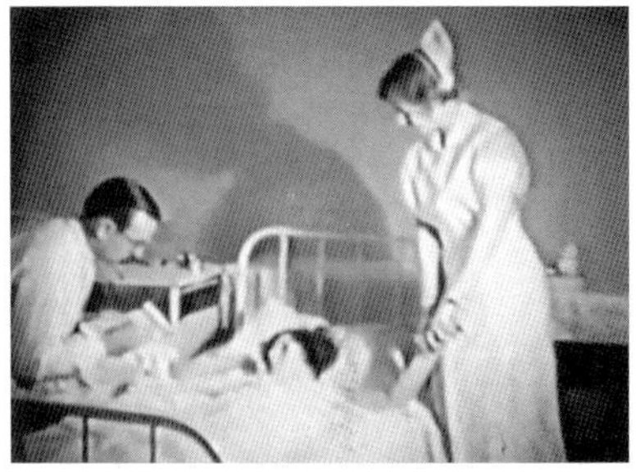

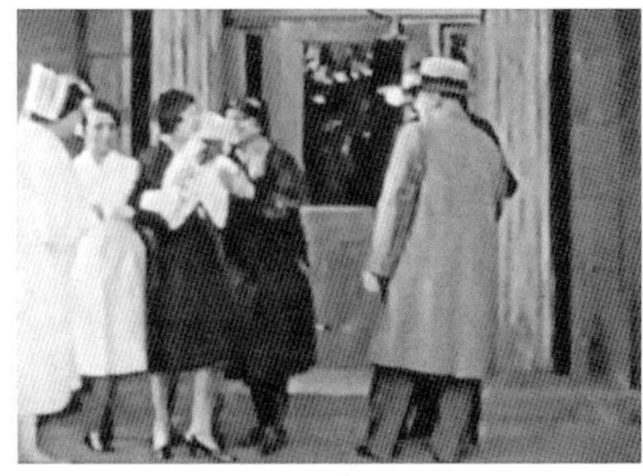

Top: *Out of the Shadows* still. *Courtesy Dennis Webster*.

Middle: Patient being seen by a doctor, from the silent film *Out of the Shadows*. *Courtesy Dennis Webster*.

Bottom: Released patient reunited with her baby, from the silent film *Out of the Shadows*. *Courtesy Dennis Webster*.

nurses change her into her patient clothing. They bring her food, and the title on screen says, "Persuading the patient to eat." The nurses try but fail at trying to feed her. "Now begins the routine examinations which all patients must receive." We see patients in bed in the receiving ward. The doctor conducts the interview. "In the search for possible causes of ill health the condition of the truth must be investigated." Mary is next placed in a dental chair while a doctor looks at her teeth. "And eye strain must not be overlooked." Then the doctor conducts an eye exam, and we see, "The danger of introducing contagious diseases into a crowded institution demands the utmost vigilance to find them early." We then see doctors and nurses taking cultures from Mary and swab her mouth. "Treatment by violet ray and other forms of electricity helps to restore the vitamins so necessary for health." We see a doctor using a stethoscope while an electrical device is placed in Mary's mouth. They then take Mary to a room of tables where she is given a pair of shaded goggles and placed on her back. They have a large lamp over her to blast ultraviolet rays. Then the next title on screen reads, "An x-ray examination is deemed necessary." In a shocking display they lie Mary on a table and slide a lead plate under her body. The nurse and doctor stand right there, unguarded from the radiation as they take the x-ray picture. Then the screen puts up the title, "The ward doctor, having completed his study of Mary Hayes' illness, brings her before the medical superintendent and staff physicians for approval of the plan of treatment he recommends."

They then bring Mary into a room full of doctors who poke, prod and question her. She is escorted out, and the scene shows the physicians looking at the x-ray. Next, "Mary receives her first visit from her husband." She sits in a chair, and her husband arrives with flowers and a hug. The title then shows, "MUST NOW MOVE ON. The annual daily arrival of new patients, necessitates, after a month, Mary's transfer from Dunham Hall, to another department of the hospital." They show a nurse escorting Mary from Dunham Hall over to Old Main, where she is placed on an elevator and taken upstairs to the packed patient ward. The film shows beds packed next to each other mere inches apart. The head nurse is unable to find her a bed, so they set one up in the hallway. Then there is a massive group of patients walking down a hall in Old Main, packed together, with the title on the screen saying, "Just one among so many - - - on the way to the crowded dining room." The hallway is jam-packed, and the screen now shows, "Crowded out and lonely."

The movie moves forward and states that it is several months later and says, "Mary is improving and has begun to renew her interest in things that

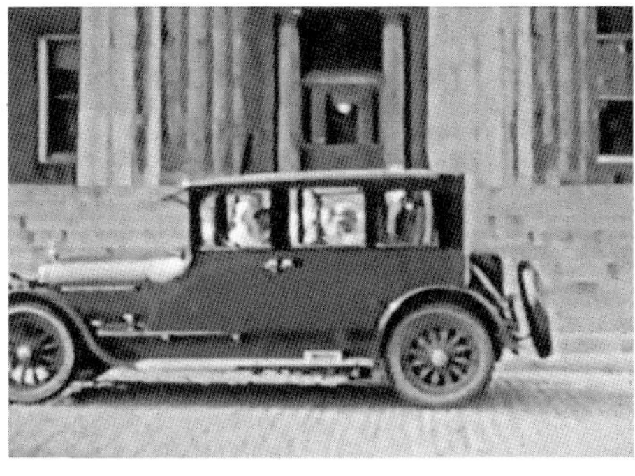

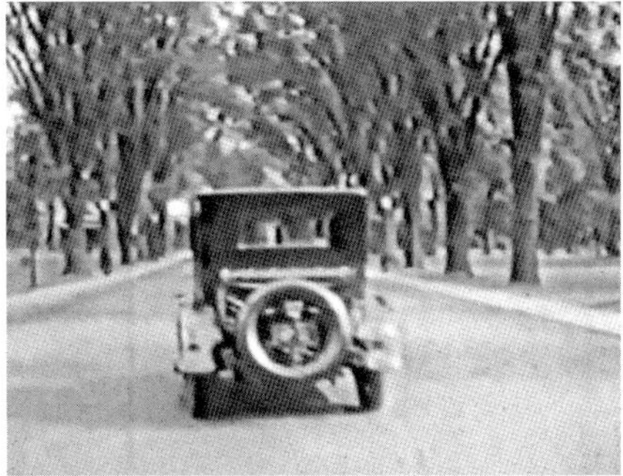

Left: Car parked ready to pick up a released patient, from the silent film *Out of the Shadows*. *Courtesy Dennis Webster.*

Right: Patient leaving Old Main, from the silent film *Out of the Shadows*. *Courtesy Dennis Webster.*

women do." They show her in a day room doing needlepoint with a group of ladies. "Busy hands drive cares away." The moral treatment seems instrumental in the improvement. Mary is then shown outside playing tennis with the title on screen, "The aid of two great specialists is called in—Dr. Exercise and Dr. Fresh Air." Next Mary is picking and smelling flowers in the hospital garden: "Day dawns—the shadows flee. Sunshine and flowers bring victory." Then Mary is getting her hair cut and nails done, "Beauty is but skin deep but the love of it comes from the heart." The doctors then meet, and they bring Mary in the room, where they look her over and discuss her status. She smiles and sits with her shoulders back. They tell her she is being discharged and a social worker will visit her periodically. We then see the nurses walking her through the pillars of Old Main, where she is handed her baby. Her husband escorts her to the waiting Model A car, and they drive away from Old Main waving a white hanky out the window of the moving automobile.

To see the silent movie, go to www.youtube.com and type "Out of the Shadows Utica State Hospital."

Willis E. Merriman, MD (1939–1946)

On November 1, 1939, Dr. Merriman took the reins as the superintendent. He had a solid background of service in the care of those afflicted with mental illness. His mentor was Dr. Charles Pilgrim, who had served under the beloved Dr. Gray. Dr. Pilgrim passed Dr. Gray's care and philosophy on to Dr. Merriman. Merriman had been the superintendent at Manhattan State Hospital for six years before coming to Old Main. He oversaw the construction of a cold storage plant, completed in 1940, that was used to store produce and for the pasteurization of the milk from the Utica State Hospital cows. With all the additions around Old Main, the total patient capacity was now 1,552, based on ward space. The daily average was an overcrowded 1,750 patients. During Dr. Merriman's tenure, the large challenge was from World War II. It caused a shortage of personnel, as many moved to assist in the war effort or went overseas to fight. By the midst of the war, the staff requirement was 500 employees. In 1943, the medical staff lost 3 men who had gone to fight; 27 officer positions at Utica State Hospital were vacant, and 38 attendants had all left to the war. Patients continued to work, with 690 of them putting in an average of 5.7 hours per day. They did everything from workshop duties to cleaning Old Main. Thus continued Dr. Brigham's moral treatment into the modern age.

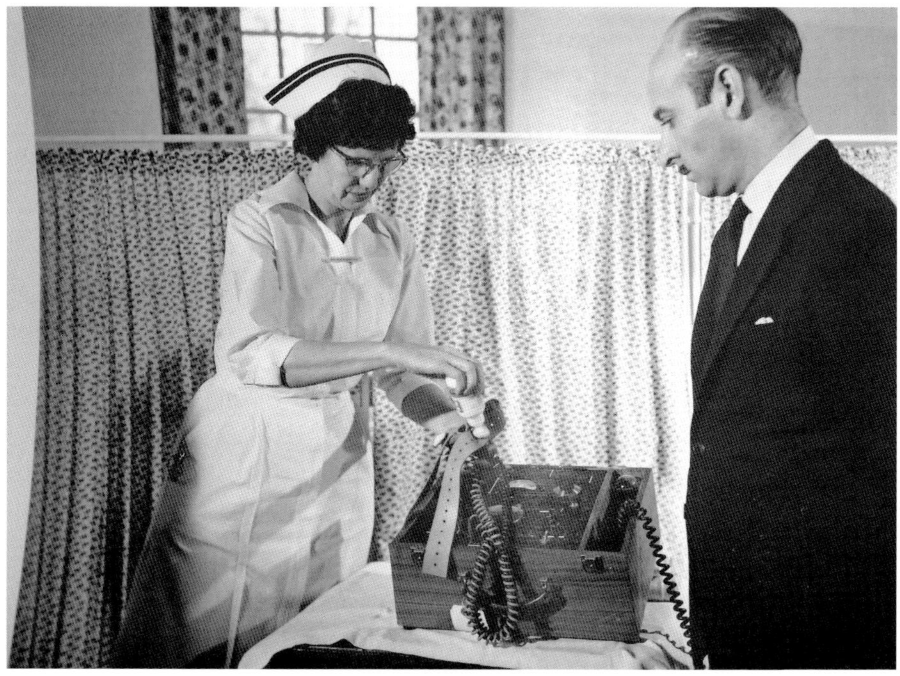

Utica State Hospital Staff demonstrate electroshock therapy machine. *New York State Archives.*

Dr. Merriman helped usher in a new modern therapeutic system for the patients that included heat therapy, chemotherapy and shock therapy. At the time, these were considered successful treatments. A popular new therapy to come to Old Main was the showing of moving pictures. This overtook all as the most popular in the hospital. These were shown in Hutchings Hall, which also hosted weekly dances. Religious services now covered all denominations and included a priest, a rabbi and a Protestant minister. By 1943, Old Main had 42,902 patients pass through its grand pillars. When it first opened, Old Main took patients from the entire state but now under Dr. Merriman, only from the five surrounding counties. Dr. Merriman oversaw Utica State Hospital during a difficult time in our country's history.

100th Anniversary Celebration

On Saturday, January 16, 1943, Utica State Hospital celebrated one hundred years of operation by having guests and exhibits. There was a large group there to celebrate a century of Old Main in Hutchings Hall. The morning session started at 10:00 a.m. and featured Whitesboro Central School Band under the leadership of Professor William A. Schnell. The dedication of the American flag was delivered by Reverend D. Charles White, Reverend Daniel B. Corrou and Rabbi S. Joshua Kohn. The guests were welcomed by superintendent Dr. Merriman with greetings by Dr. William Tiffany, commissioner of the New York State Department of Mental Hygiene. The following lecture was on shock therapy delivered by Dr. W.W. Wright, superintendent of Marcy State Hospital. In the lower floor, there was a demonstration from the school of nursing on showing the old and new methods of applying a sedative pack. The occupational therapy department was showing off the preindustrial work done at Utica State Hospital. There was music by Utica Free Academy A Cappella Choir led by Marcella Lally, displays by the Utica Public Library and the Utica Public Schools. Historical relics on display included a vast array of restraints such as the Utica crib. By 1942, there were 108,399 people with mental health disabilities under care in New York State facilities.

Arthur W. Pense, MD (1946–1948)
Harold A. Pooler, MD (1948–1949)
Francis J. O'Neill, MD (1949–1951)

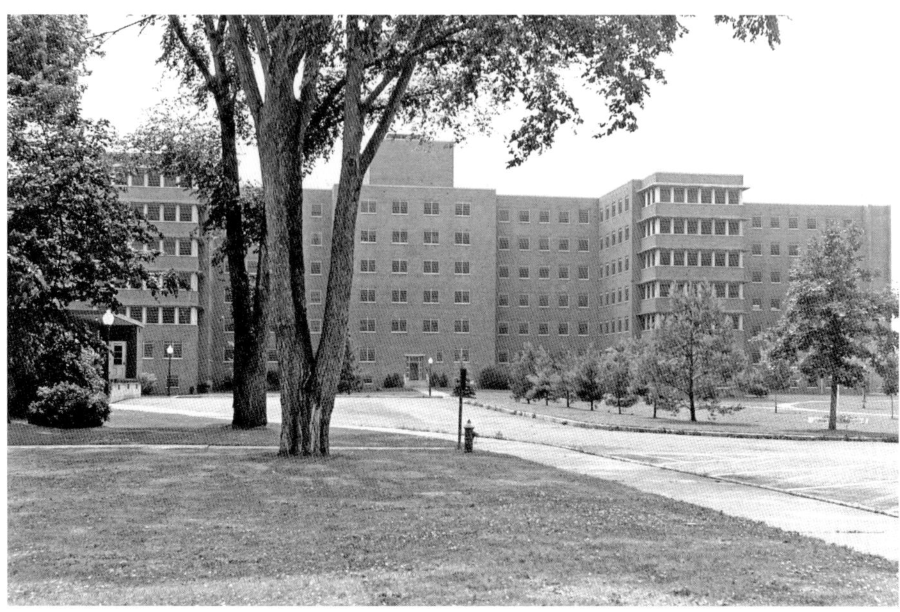

Brigham Building on the Old Main campus. It expanded patient care and opened in 1954. *New York State Archives*.

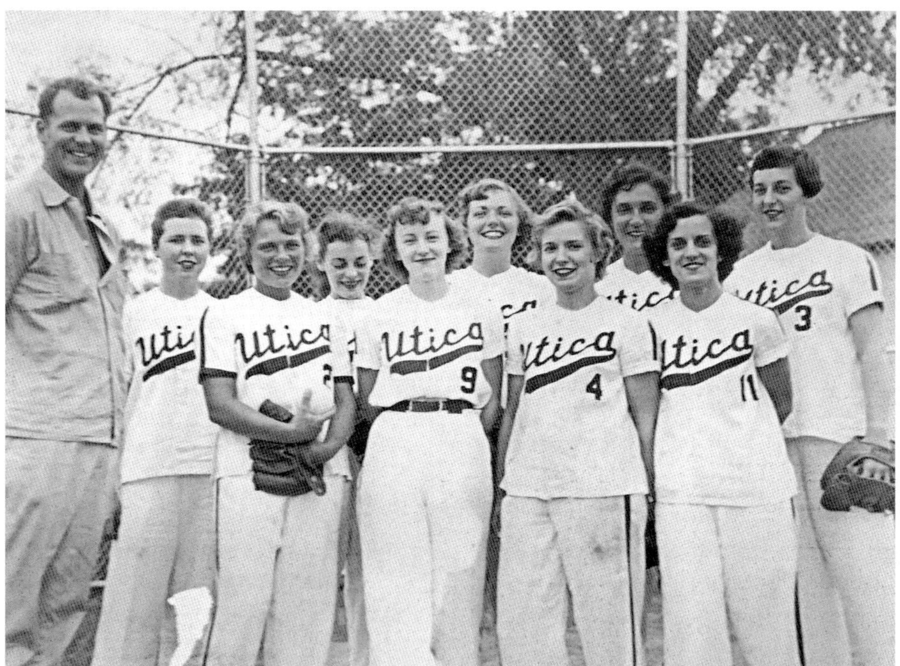

Utica State Hospital staff softball team. *New York State Archives*.

The next three superintendents of Utica State Hospital had short tenures with very little major advancements in patient care or construction projects. Automotive equipment was now being used to assist on the hospital farm, but the treatment plans still had some of the patients picking vegetables. The barn on the farm was no longer deemed necessary and had been converted to a bowling alley in 1949. These doctors would be in the midst of new forms of treatment—mainly electroshock therapy and lobotomies. Eventually, lobotomies would be phased out as better treatments became available, but electroshock therapy would stay in practice for decades. Both tend to be viewed with a modern eye as not proper; however, physicians at the time were practicing modern methodology to treat and possibly cure those who suffered with mental illness.

Bascomb B. Young, MD (1951–1959)

Dr. Young took over as superintendent of Old Main when the farm was transitioning away and land transfers were happening. In 1953, the hospital's dairy cows and horses were moved to other mental health facilities still farming. In 1954, farmland was transferred to Utica College, Zion Lutheran Church, St. Luke's Hospital and the City of Utica. Utica State Hospital had been renting land on French Road that was sold to General Electric, which erected a factory on the property. Dr. Young still had a vegetable garden at Old Main even though the facility was no longer in the farming business. Dr. Young ushered in a new era of drug treatments at the facility. For the first time in history, proper drugs had been discovered to assist in some forms of mania. A big move was the ending of locked doors and beginning an open-door policy where patients could move about the hospital with freedom. Dr. Young oversaw the construction of the Brigham Building on the Old Main campus, with the structure opening in 1955. The building was to help relieve overcrowding. In 1957, labor improvements included implementing the forty-hour work week

Martin Lazar, MD (1959–1963)

Dr. Lazar took over as superintendent from Dr. Young right when Old Main, and the entire Utica State Hospital, was at its peak with 2,534 patients. In order to alleviate the overcrowding and progress at the same

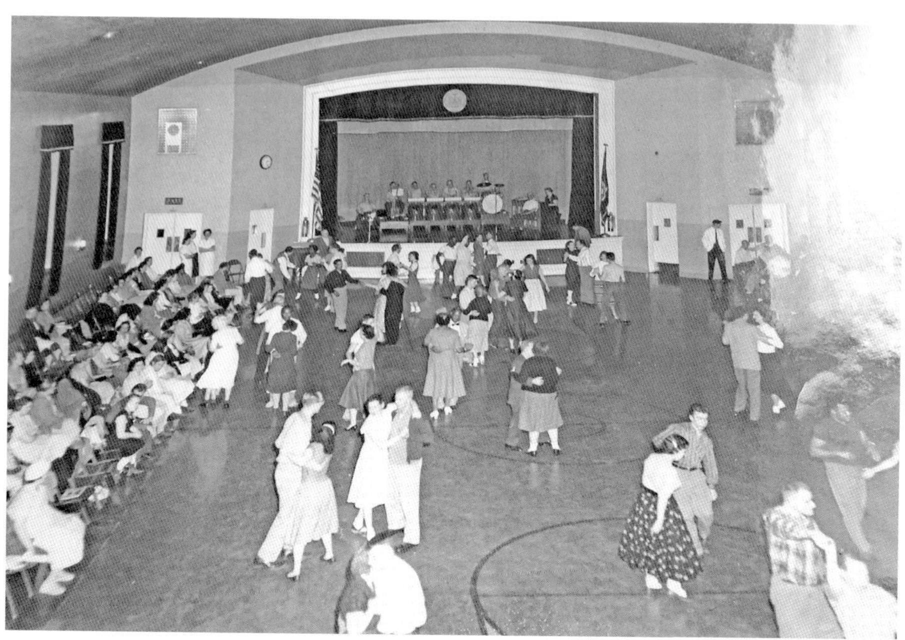

Utica State Hospital patient dance. *New York State Archives.*

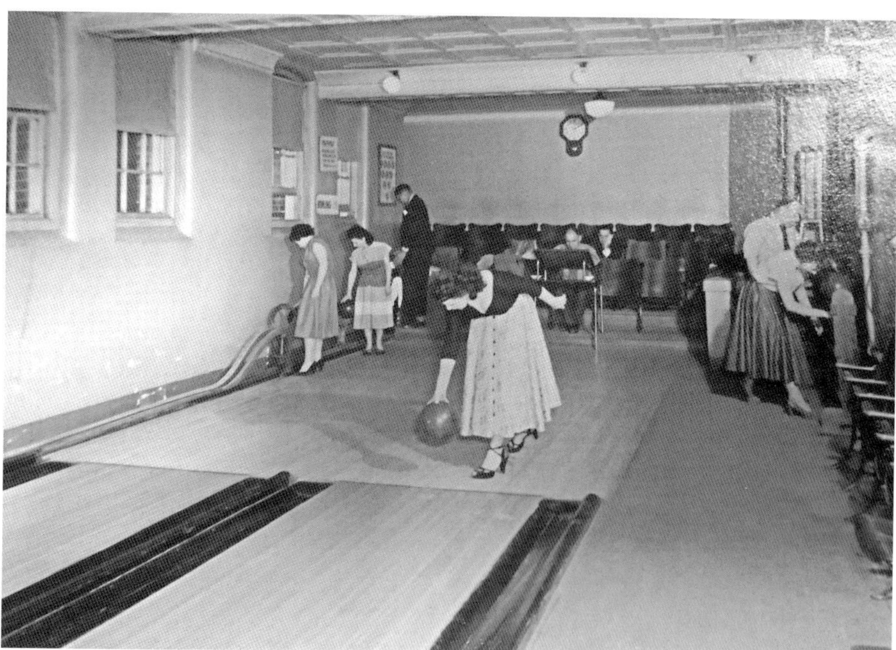

Bowling alley at Utica State Hospital. *New York State Archives.*

time, Dr. Lazar started a community program where more patients were released and integrated in what was referred to as "normalization." The institutional look was being replaced with a remodel that made it more home-like and private to the patients. A new narcotic unit was opened in 1962 to treat those with drug mania and addiction. This unit would operate until 1968. The patients and staff enjoyed working for Dr. Lazar, who expanded patient activities with bowling leagues, softball teams and increased field trips. He also encouraged the patients to remodel their wings, with many painting the walls a multitude of colors. Religious services increased, and he oversaw the addition and grand opening of the synagogue for Jewish patients and their families.

George Volow, MD (1963–1976)

Dr. Volow took over as superintendent at Utica State Hospital in 1963 and would serve thirteen years in the position. He took over at a crucial time in American history, as President Kennedy had just been assassinated. Dr. Volow addressed the patients and staff, stating he hoped the president's spirit and ideals would carry them throughout their lives. He established an intensive retreatment unit at Dunham Hall in order to provide rehabilitation and intervention to a chosen group of chronic patients. The patient care was then broken up from unit names to those after the county of patient origin. This kept patients from the same counties together and attempted to create a tighter unit between the patients and the staff. Southside, Northside and Admissions were replaced with Fulton, Montgomery, Saratoga, Schenectady and Utica units. Social service agencies from each county listed would form a strong bond with the unit. Reintegration into their home communities began to thin the patient population at Old Main. More and more patients were being sent to Marcy State Hospital, yet Utica still had a strong base of care. Dr. Volow undertook the creation of a sheltered workshop in 1972 that created paid work for the patients. The workshop was located on the second floor of Old Main, across from the Jewish Chapel. They manufactured goods and worked on subcontracts for local businesses. In 1974, Old Main would undergo its last name change when Utica State Hospital became the Utica Psychiatric Center. Talks of Marcy or Utica closing or a merger had begun. This name change on May 23, 1974, would occur right at the end of Dr. Volow's tenure. Old Main also achieved national recognition on October 26, 1971, when it was placed in the National Register of Historic Places.

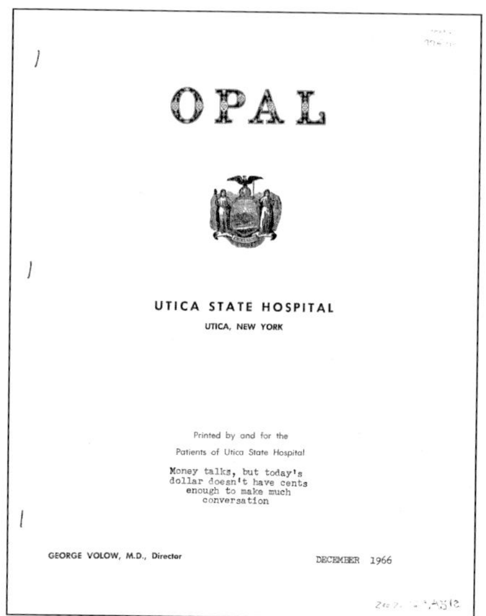

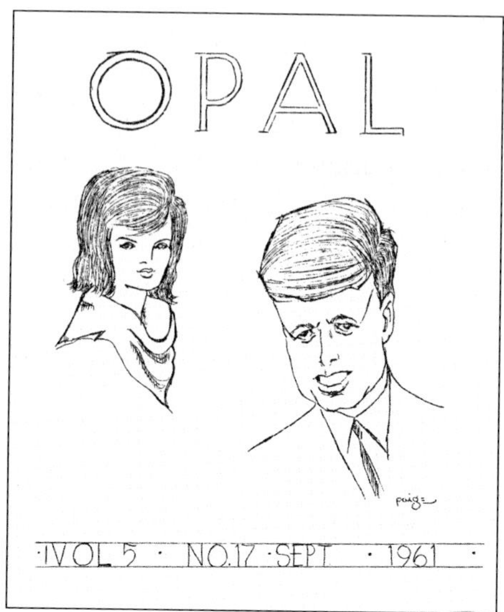

Left: Mid twentieth-century cover of the *Opal*. *Oneida County History Center*.

Right: Front cover art of President Kennedy and first lady by Robert Paige. *Oneida County History Center*.

The Opal Resurrected

In 1957, the *Opal* came back as a quarterly publication. The newly resurrected *Opal* would run longer than the original and was published until 1976. The big difference with this version would be that it featured much more about the staff and much less patient writing. It would still have short stories and some poems but not the same amount. It seems this was more for internal use than the original *Opal* sold to the public had been. The following tidbits were featured in the following *Opal* issues:

March 1957. This issue was published by the Patients' Society. The George Alder Bloomer Laboratory, started in 1920, performed 91,042 tests in the previous year, including outside testing for Uticans. Animal testing was being done on guinea pigs, rabbits and mice. They tested for tuberculosis and conducted pregnancy tests for women using the rabbits. The Choraleers, a choir made up of men and women patients of Utica State Hospital, performed many times in Utica and appeared on television twice. The group was directed by Mrs. Michael Levine. Old Main hosted a wonderful rendition of *Oklahoma!* performed by the patients. Religion appeared in the new version of the *Opal* with an essay about liberty written by Rabbi I. David Essrig. The Occupational Therapy (OT) department advertised patient-made rugs, a popular item that always sold out. The Utica Public Library sent a librarian regularly to Old Main to distribute books from a large rolling oak cart. The hobby shop continued to be popular with the men, and they made all kinds of goods for sale and use. Some donated wood needed to be sanded and stripped, and many enjoyed the process. Recreations listed in the *Opal* were card parties, dances and afternoon teas. Sports were part of this program, with bowling being popular. A bowling tournament was held between two wards: North Side from Old Main versus the Brigham Building Stars. Old Main won the tournament, led by patient F.D., who rolled a 206. The Old Main crew was hoping to get a bowling match against the patient bowling team from Marcy State Hospital.

September 1961. The cover featured a hand-drawn portrait of President John F. Kennedy and First Lady Jacqueline Kennedy done by Robert Paige. Inside was a poem dedicated to their daughter, Caroline, written by Father Owen McEnaney:

"To Caroline"

Kneel Down by your bed, little Caroline
And clasp your hands in prayer,
And close your eyes as you whisper
To someone whose truly there.

Please take care of my Daddy,
He's President, God, you know…
Help him do the very best job…
Tell him the way to go.

He's head over millions of people
Whose lives are in his hands. . .
Help him to keep them peaceful and free
And proud of our wonderful land.

And God, take care of my Mommy
And my brother, Baby John;
Make us a family the whole world will love…
And you'll always smile upon.

A nice thank-you from the patients went out to the Utica State Hospital repair shop and its two employees, Carl Hasler and Jack Phillips, who had just repaired the television. The men also repaired all the radios and phonographs at the hospital. The Hoe and Hope Garden Club had a show at the hospital. A weight-lifting class had been started along with a garment manufacturing class, both of which expanded recreation options for the patients. A group of patients was taken to the Utica Memorial Auditorium to watch a wrestling show.

DECEMBER 1961. Anna K. Lee retired after thirty years as the secretary to the superintendent. She served under six superintendents during her long tenure. The party was held at Twin Ponds. A copy of the previous *Opal* was sent to President Kennedy and a thank-you letter sent in return from Ralph Dungan, special agent to the president. The recreational activities included pinochle, bowling, basketball, movies and meetings of the "Golden Age Club" for patients sixty years or older. The Christmas party included a show, a dance and carols sung by the Student Nurses. The patients' Community Store had a holiday sale that included patient-made Christmas cards, wrapping paper, costume jewelry and many other items, from makeup to cigarettes and a line of pipes. The Narcotic Unit was opening with patients both self-admitted and court-ordered. The "Magic Trunk," located on the South Side wing Ward 16, was filled with donations from local churches and individuals. The trunk, overseen by patient Miss K, was a room of donated clothing and goods for patients to go through and help themselves. Most were patients who didn't have relatives or visitors. The patients enjoyed going out into the community to see the Shrine Circus and the finals of the Barber Shop Quartet competition. The patients on the North Side wing were pleased to be able to repaint all the rooms in a variety of colors. The Hobby Shop was flooded with orders for their hand-made wood goods. The South Side reported a stray cat that had become a welcome visitor to the patients, but a skunk hanging around had them turning their noses up.

MARCH 1962. A tribute to John Glenn's space flight around the globe was written with great joy and pride. The writer asked, "Did you know Colonel Glenn saw three sunrises and three sunsets?" Rabbi Essrig, the Jewish chaplain, wrote an essay on why Passover is significant to freedom. Chaplain Anthony and Father Stack wrote some Easter prayers. The Drama Class, under the direction of Gloria Cohen, was auditioning patients to be in a new comedy performance. The men of the North Side had oiled wooden items and burned Mickey Mouse characters into many of the wooden pieces. The *Opal* staff held a session on creative writing with their fellow patients. The newsletter continued to be printed and distributed by the hospital patients.

June 1962. On Wednesday, May 2, the synagogue was dedicated in the name of Dr. A.J. Goldstein. It was located on the second floor of the South Side of Old Main. The first services were attended by many patients who heard Rabbi Essrig. The Hobby Shop made and painted wooden fish that hung in the dining hall. Neisner's Store, Genesee Street, Utica, donated enough Easter candy for four hundred patients. Larry's Bakery, Varick Street, Utica, donated enough fancy baked goods for four hundred patients. A group of twenty-five patients went to the Utica Zoo, where they delighted in the gorilla that threw carrots at them. Another group of patients was able to go to the Oneida County Airport, where they were able to see the hangar and some planes. Patients enjoyed the outdoors, as they pitched in to assist the grounds department in the beautification of the hospital landscape. The new baseball season had started, so patients were enjoying the games on the television and radio. The sewing group from the senior center at Munson Williams Proctor Institute came and made drapes and other items with the patients. Fourteen patients took and completed an advanced first-aid class. The theater group was looking for patients interested in acting, singing and dancing. Some activities included a bingo party picnic, the M&S Patient Band concert, a block dance, an employee softball game and name that tune.

For the rest of its run, the *Opal* cover would feature the New York State Crest on the front. No more patient art.

September 1962. Patients enjoyed a trip to the Oriskany Battlefield and Summit Park, where they had a picnic lunch. The patients gathered with male employees to discuss fishing, with one picture of a humungous northern pike taken from the St. Lawrence River by one employee. Due to a new planer machine, the wood shop added manufacturing picture frames to its list of wood goods. The School of Nursing held its graduation ceremony at Proctor High School on September 12 from 2:00 to 4:00 p.m. Patients and employees at a recent blood drive donated thirty-nine pints of blood.

December 1962. A new parking lot was constructed at the rear of the Brigham Building. Parking rules would be strictly enforced by the hospital police. Safety rules prohibited electric lights on all Utica State Hospital

Christmas trees. Patients went on a trip to Hamilton College and a hockey game at the Clinton Arena. A French class and typing class were added to the writing group's activities. Patients were selling their handmade holiday cards. Sunday organ recitals had recently started with much fun by all.

March 1963. The Shoe Hospital at Utica State Hospital was run by William Orsomarso, or "Bill," as everyone called him. He had performed emergency shoe repairs at the hospital since 1948. The patients enjoyed their trips to Bill and his Shoe Hospital, where he greeted them with a smile and handcrafted repaired footwear. The American Legion Posts from Frankfort, Ilion and Mohawk, as well as their ladies' auxiliary, hosted a party for hospital patients in January, held at the Crowley-Barnum Post in Mohawk. The Mohigans provided the music, with additional entertainment by the Melo-Tones. There were door prizes, cigarettes and a dance contest. Fun was had by all. The retired teachers association sent teachers to assist teenage patients in their studies in order to improve their scores in mathematics, English, science and social studies. The teacher volunteers were greeted with much appreciation.

June 1963. In this edition were lots of well wishes from patients and staff, as Dr. Lazar resigned as superintendent. The Utica State Hospital library increased its holdings in the previous year by almost one thousand books. Green benches were placed under trees around the hospital campus so patients could enjoy reading outside. Recent volunteer groups came from the American Legions from Sherrill, Mohawk, Ilion and Frankfort, Pat Sovicki Dance Group, Anthony McKenos String Ensemble, Local Musicians Union, the Genetaska from Whitesboro, Seed and Weed Garden Club, Town and Country Garden Club and the New Hartford Garden Club.

September 1963. This issue offered greetings to the new director, Dr. George Volow. The South Side Patients Society in Old Main hosted a welcome tea for Dr. Volow and his wife. Falling plaster from the ceilings did not land on any patients or staff. The maintenance department fixed the damages. The Floral Art group held its annual display with the theme "Autumn Harvest Crowns the Earth." The employee softball league team ended its season with a 9-7 record. J. White led the team with a .555 average, and L. Milucci had the most hits with 21.

December 1963. The safety department supervisor attended a civilian defense seminar on managing a fallout shelter with a training exercise to follow for a two-hundred-bed shelter in case of nuclear war. Many patients were able to go home to their families for Thanksgiving dinner. The patient bowling teams were the Mets, Yogi Spares, the Spares and Ten Pins. The league title went to the Mets with a record of 19-5. Patient J.K. from ward 11 had the highest patient bowling average with a 172.

MARCH 1964. Ed Zucker, painter in charge of the paint shop, received a certificate of merit from the Civil Service Commission plus one hundred dollars cash bonus. He won this award by improving the Ransburg Painting Process used at Old Main. The entire Utica State Hospital campus had a total population of employees and patients of 3,500. The French class learned new songs popular in France. The safety department warned all employees and patients not to dispose of their cigarette butts in the garbage receptacles. Fire was a serious danger, so they were asked to put butts out in water. The community store was selling Easter corsages for fifty cents and cards for five cents, along with Easter eggs, boxed candy and other items. Friends from the Zonta Club in Utica visited and performed a fashion show for the patients. The Foot Hill Council of the Girl Scouts donated Christmas decorations. Volunteers donated ten thousand hours of service to Utica State Hospital in 1963.

JUNE 1964. The Model Airplane Club was looking for members. Robert Shockley was appointed pharmacist at Utica State Hospital and Dr. Joseph A. Gambacorta dentist. The peach tree on ward 15 was bearing fruit for the first time. Night baseball games started.

SEPTEMBER 1964. The new Intensive Retreatment Unit opened at Dunham Hall. A fire drill was held, and pandemonium ruled as the halls became congested, including the arrival of off-duty employees. As a result, the safety department would be forming a hospital fire brigade. A safer and cleaner milk delivery system was being piloted at Old Main with new milk dispensers. This eliminated pouring milk from can to can, which had cleanliness issues. Father John Stack, the hospital's Catholic priest, recently aced the thirteenth hole at the Yahundasis Golf Club. He shot the hole in one using an eight iron on the 138-yard hole. A documentary film was shot at Old Main by the Civil Service Employee Association of New York State. It was to promote careers in New York State and featured footage from the hospital nursing staff.

DECEMBER 1964. Alec Dana was teaching very popular dance classes at the Brigham Building. The annual Christmas dance held at Old Main featured the music of the Laurence Luizzi Orchestra. Coffee, punch and sandwiches were served. The annual Halloween game party once again proved to be most popular among the patients and staff. The Utica State Hospital Auxiliary donated sixty-three sets of china dishes to the South Side ward.

MARCH 1965. The Magic Trunk celebrated two years of operation. Many from the community donated to the Magic Trunk, and 223 patients used the trunk in 1964. The Book Review Group was now meeting and looking for members. The Utica State Auxiliary was looking for members. The dues were one dollar per year, and members partook in numerous volunteer activities at Old Main and other Utica State Hospital buildings. The hospital Chorus Line got new red shirts and white blouses. They would be proudly worn at their next performance. Burton C. Tyeick, sixty-one, recently passed away. He had been the Utica State Hospital barber since 1928, with thirty-seven years of dedicated haircutting service.

JUNE 1965. Many patients from the South Side enjoyed a trip to the West End Brewery. Three patients recently took and passed their high school equivalency exams. The employees and patients undertook a campaign to collect five thousand tea bag tags in order to acquire a seeing-eye dog for a local blind girl. The patients planted a new geranium bed, started their softball season and went fishing with new gear that had been donated by Neisner's and Woolworths in Utica. The employees started a T.O.P.S. (take off the pounds sensibly) weight loss club. The Utica State Bowling Team made up of employees won the league title. They bowled at Bliss Alleys, now called Seafare, in Whitesboro. The annual bake sale and open house was a success. The summer recreation for the patients included softball, miniature golf, downtown movies, picnics, a fishing trip and swimming.

SEPTEMBER 1965. The final phase of the fallout shelters was complete with the filling of 1,200 barrels of water. In a nod back to the original *Opal*, Dr. Gray announced that the number of subscribers had exceeded two thousand. A book jacket design contest was underway, with patients designing covers for their favorite books in the Old Main library.

DECEMBER 1965. The safety department reminded all Utica State Hospital employees and patients to get away from radioactive fallout from a nuclear strike by following the fallout shelter signs posted in all the buildings. A program, *Working Smarter and Not Harder*, was delivered to all patients and employees engaged in the workshops.

MARCH 1966. A snow emergency forced the staff and nurses to work seven straight shifts without a break. Dr. Volow, superintendent of Utica State Hospital, wrote a thank-you letter to the dedicated staff. This was the legendary Utica area "blizzard of 66" that many recall most fondly. The Utica War Memorial hosted the Clinton Comets, with many of the hospital patients enjoying the hockey action.

JUNE 1966. The community store offered printed hankies for the ladies at twenty-five cents each. Ladies from Ward 19 enjoyed visiting Kernan School and meeting all the students and teachers. Old Main got a "best dressed" award for the new colors in the painted rooms. The Utica State Hospital Golf League started the season at Hidden Valley Golf Course in Whitesboro. Dozens of employees from all departments were in the league.

SEPTEMBER 1966. A new five-speaker stereophonic system was installed in the woodworking shop. Munson Williams Proctor Institute accepted one of the lady patient's oil paintings for its summer 1966 show. Prayers were said for all the boys for a safe return from Vietnam. The Utica Dog Obedience Club held a dog show on the front lawn in front of Old Main. Patients and staff enjoyed the many types of pooches. The hospital grounds now had 51 acres of land, 500 lawn benches, 12 picnic tables and 30 trash cans. The patients had for their use two volleyball courts, a basketball court, two horseshoe pits, and five holes for pitch and putt golf. There were 12 flower beds, a vegetable garden, 2,600 trees of 52 varieties and 1,600 shrubs of 27 varieties. The 300 rose bushes added extra beauty.

DECEMBER 1966. A Christmas performance by Bill McHugo's dancing school proved to be most popular. A billiards tournament was underway. The patients wanted the readers of the *Opal* to know how much tender loving care they received from the staff. The safety department was pleased at the results of the latest fire drill, as all responded in quick and efficient manner. The Utica Fire Department assisted the fire drill. The safety department suggested that everyone purchase their loved ones a fire extinguisher as a Christmas present. The woodshop made several wooden drop boxes for the patients to leave their library books.

Spring 1969. In a staff interview, it was revealed that the superintendent, Dr. Volow, liked to smoke American cigars. He preferred Cubans, but they were hard to get. He was also an accomplished violin player and played the viola in the Utica Symphony Orchestra. Dr. Volow revealed that he felt Old Main would be retired as a place for the mentally ill soon. He said the side wings should be torn down and the remaining structure, the front with its iconic pillars, remain and become a museum that houses medical journals from around the world.

Part III

Utica Psychiatric Center (1974–1978)

Nelson Sanchez, MD (1976–1977)

Dr. Sanchez took over as the superintendent of Utica Psychiatric Hospital right as the names changed at both Marcy and Utica. Dr. Sanchez was the superintendent of Marcy Psychiatric Center and now added Utica to his duties. The two facilities retained their separate identities and independence of each other. A controversial decision had been made in 1977, when those deemed criminally insane were transferred from the New York State Department of Corrections to the Office of Mental Health. These patients would be placed at Marcy, but if they required surgical services, they'd be sent to Utica. This arrangement would last for two years; afterward, patients would be sent to local hospitals.

Richard M. Heath (1977–1992)

Heath would be both the first and the last. He would be the first nonmedical doctor to supervise Old Main in its grand history. He would also be the last supervisor to serve underneath the historic structure, as Old Main closed after 135 years. The doors were closed to patients and locked to the

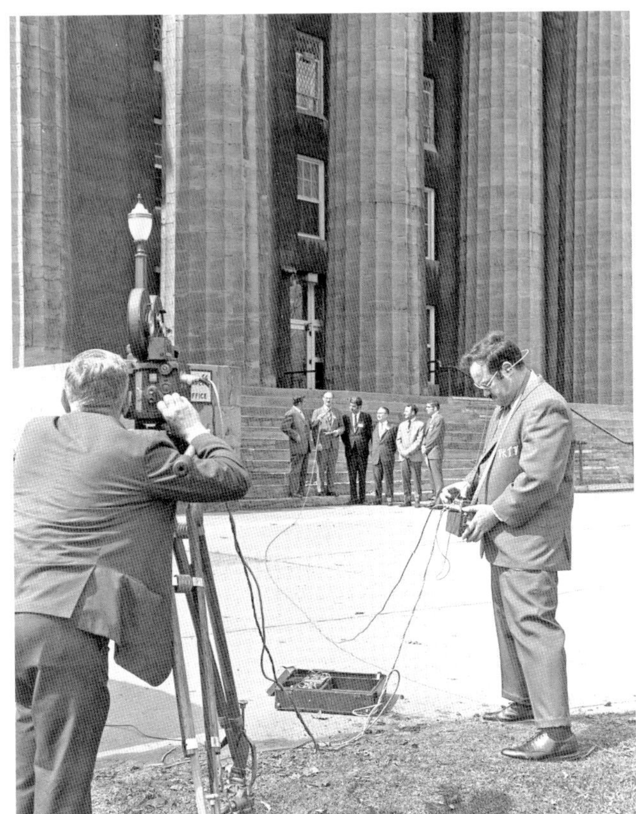

Right: Utica television station WKTV reporting from the grand pillars of Old Main. *New York State Archives*.

Below: Plaque affixed to the front column by the entrance to the Old Main campus. *Courtesy Dennis Webster*.

UTICA STATE HOSPITAL
1843
THE FIRST INSTITUTION BUILT
BY THE STATE OF NEW YORK
FOR THE CARE AND TREATMENT
OF THE MENTALLY ILL.

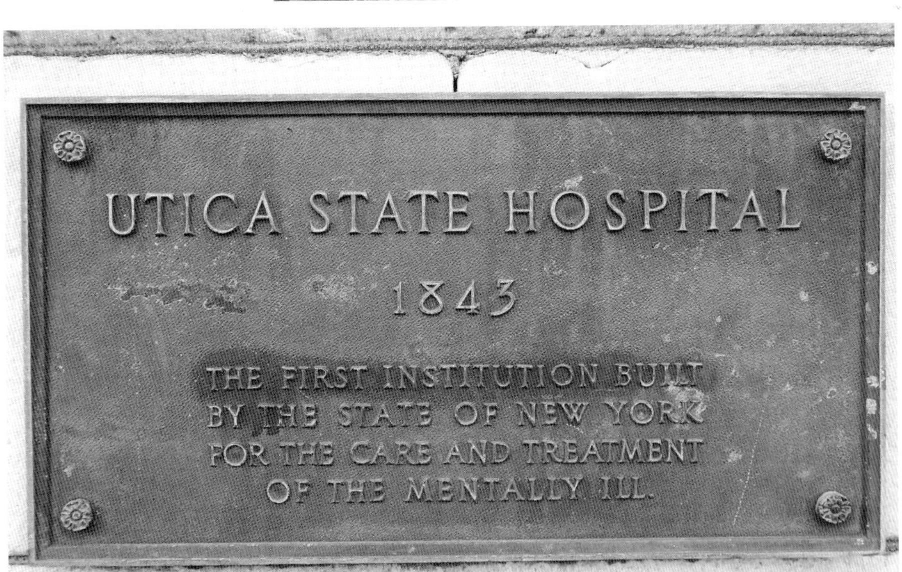

public on September 28, 1978. The building had been deemed a safety hazard and too expensive to fix. All the patients were transferred to other buildings on the Utica campus.

Post-Closure Psychiatric Care in the Mohawk Valley

Old Main shut its doors; however, the Utica Psychiatric Center campus remained active, with psychiatric care still taking place on the Utica campus with a smattering of buildings and services. The facility is now called the Mohawk Valley Psychiatric Center. You can see some activity at Old Main with a New York State record-keeping operation, and there are still cars and people working on the campus. The moral treatment started by Dr. Brigham in Utica 172 years ago still exists in patient care for those with mental disabilities.

Haunted Old Main

There is no doubt that the single place in New York State, and nationally, that is on the wish list of every ghost hunter, paranormal enthusiast or curiosity seeker is the Old Main building that was the Lunatic Asylum at Utica when it first opened in 1843. Could it be the foreboding pillars that greet you as you come up the main road to the psychiatric center? Or the tall gray walls with metal mesh in the windows? From the outside, it *looks* haunted. Many staff members who worked there in the 1970s, when the name was Utica Psychiatric Center, claim to have heard entities walking around the abandoned floors or the spirits of the dead roaming the tunnels and basement, dragging chains behind them for all eternity. Len Bragg, who was a student nurse many years after Old Main closed, recalled a haunting experience. The nursing students were given a guided tour of Old Main, and Len felt a dark, foreboding atmosphere as soon as the group walked between the pillars and inside the abandoned building. The group went deep inside the asylum, and he felt the hair on the back of his neck raise, as somebody not of this earth was with them. It was dark, but the minimal light allowed Len to see an apparition moving down

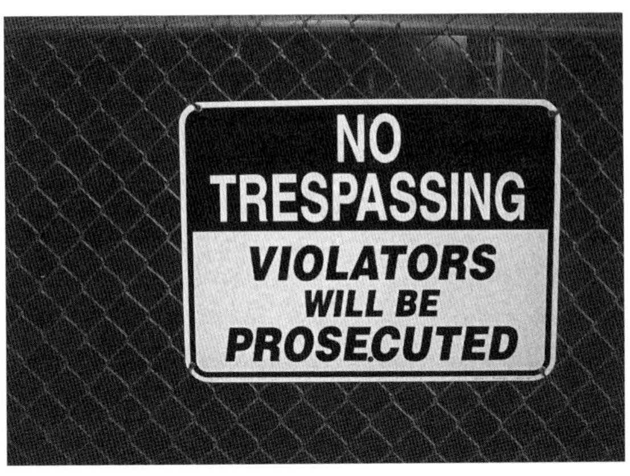

Old Main is off-limits to the curious. *Courtesy Dennis Webster.*

the hall. Many years later, Len was employed at the Brigham Building, on the Utica Psychiatric Center campus, and would return with a group to once again tour the abandoned Old Main. Upon entering the darkened halls, he once again caught a glimpse of a ghost and felt the presence. Len has been a paranormal investigator for over forty years and currently is a member of the Ghost Seekers of Central New York. Bernadette Peck, lead paranormal investigator and founder of the Ghost Seekers, has long had a fascination with Old Main. In 2013, she led her group on a ghost hunt around the perimeter of the building. Visitors are not granted access inside, but even with this limited access, the Ghost Seekers acquired electronic voice phenomenon (EVPs) and captured ectoplasm streaks and spirit lights emanating from the windows, but the best piece of evidence was captured on night vision video camera. It was a ghost walking across a window on the second floor. "It's rare to capture a moving ghost on film," said Bernadette. The investigation was late on a Saturday night, so there was no mortal person inside. The New York State records room on the first floor does not operate late on Saturday nights. From viewing the footage, you can see it is a shadow person and not a solid person looking out the window. "You can feel the sadness from the spirits," said Bernadette. "There are trapped souls inside Old Main." Back in 2003, the Paranormal & Ghost Society entered Old Main and stayed inside for only one hour, but the results were thrilling. They heard footsteps, recorded voices and captured droves of spirit lights and a large twisting ectoplasm. Their team witnessed this ectoplasm twirling like a cyclone that spun down the hall. "Old Main is absolutely haunted," said Paranormal & Ghost Society founder Lord Rick Rowe.

The paranormal occurrences started right from the beginning, when the facility was only sixteen years into its existence. The building was then the Lunatic Asylum at Utica, and the patients wrote, edited and published their own monthly periodical called the *Opal*. Within the pages of the volume published in 1859, an article written by an unnamed ex-patient described the ghost of a claimed "Seminole-Indian extinguisher" or self-proclaimed Indian killer walking the halls of the eastern wing, knocking on walls and doors at all hours of the night, keeping the patients awake. The passage reads, "We hate to throw aside an unfinished plan into the 'dust pan of oblivion,' as Dow, Jr., expresses it; and even though we should hear of the sudden death of the Seminole Indian-extinguisher, we are not sure but his ghost would appear with credentials knocking for admittance at the 'eastern' Opalian gate. We fear his ghost. He can amuse if he gets in the mood. We think he has not been entertaining thus far." The writer goes on to state that the ghost of the Indian killer was a man most insane when committed and tends to conduct practical jokes and pranks on the living. It is important to note that Old Main is not open to the public, and a permanent fence encircles the building to keep the curious public and ghost hunters at bay. Signs warn away the curious.

What Is to Happen to Old Main?

Brian Howard, former executive director of the Oneida County History Center, provided the following when asked about the fate of Old Main:

> *The venerable structure we know as "Old Main" is of vital importance to the story of the greater Mohawk Valley. This is much more than just another old building—it is a structure of national significance, architecturally and historically. Unfortunately for the building, it has also outlived its originally intended purpose. Old Main is one of the earliest, largest, and most significant examples of Greek Revival architecture in the United States. Its central pillars, eight feet in diameter at the base, anchor an imposing façade that is sure to impress any first-time visitor to the facility. There is a reason that it is on the National Register of Historic Places—a designation that it first achieved over four decades ago. It is a shame to see this grand structure as it stands in 2015. The asylum's days as a clinic and healing center are long gone and it is a harbinger of another era, when institutionalization was standard treatment for the mentally ill. Several cracked windows, sags and stained*

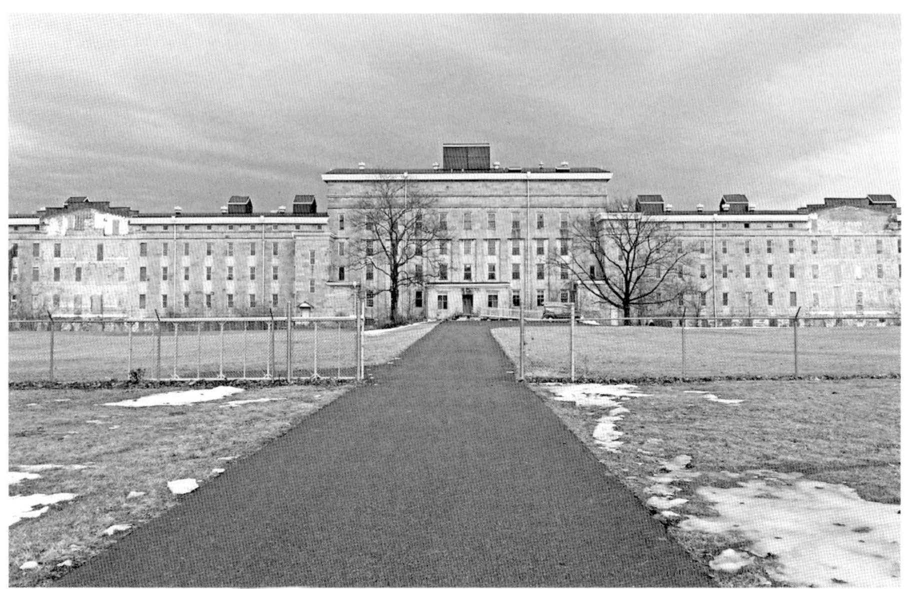

Rear entrance to Old Main. *Courtesy Jeff Berman.*

masonry belie its age. Left untreated, the leaking roof will lead to bigger problems that may be impossible to address. Short of demolition, it is going to take a massive investment to ensure its long-term viability.

Its Continuing Appeal

So, why does Old Main generate such a passionate following? A lot of it has to do with it being a tangible link to Utica's "glory days" of the late 19th and early 20th centuries. This booming factory town was a cradle of national political power during the Industrial Age. Thanks to the Erie Canal and an extensive rail system, this was also a transportation crossroads and a center of commerce. As a pioneering psychiatric care facility, the New York State Lunatic Asylum was a vital part of the region's progressive, forward-looking persona. Even after a century, letting go of this identity can be an awful hard thing to do.

Much of Old Main's appeal revolves around the public's enduring fascination with mental illness. Especially for those who have no personal connection to it, the idea of madness has an alluring, dare I say…perverse

(?)…attraction. Kind of like driving slow past an auto accident. Hollywood has capitalized on this for decades; Norman Bates in Psycho *and Michael Myers from* Halloween *are just two examples for whom mental illness was at the root of their character. I think the idea of having a "creepy old insane asylum" in town appeals to this base curiosity—it's the fear of the unknown. More recently, the groundswell of interest in the paranormal has put Old Main on the map of ghost hunters near and far. Again, the Hollywood factor comes in to play here. What better place to investigate than an abandoned facility that has been described more than once as a "house of horrors" for those interned there? Whether one is a believer or a skeptic, there is no doubt that this aspect has brought thousands to its doors every time a public tour is conducted.*

The Future

Too much has changed in the field of psychiatry to ever consider using Old Main again for the treatment of the mentally ill. Those days are gone. But the fact that so much pioneering mental health work occurred there, alone makes this grand building worthy of preservation. Not to mention its architectural significance or its relevance to Utica's city history. Old Main's story—Utica's story—is not unique. The northeast United States is saturated with huge structures, built for another time and which are standing today without a purpose. Many will be demolished. Some will be saved. Old Main should fall in the latter category; it is too much a part of this area's story to fall to the wrecking ball. The key is adaptive reuse.

For years, ideas have been bandied about with regard to repurposing Old Main. Turning it into a "national mental health museum," as has been proposed over the years, is an effort that I feel is neither realistic nor sustainable. This building's story needs to be preserved, of course, but not in the guise of a cultural heritage facility. What needs to happen is for a viable business plan to be developed, perhaps a private-public partnership, or a city-state partnership, to bring revenue-generating activities on site. The state is already using the building for records storage; perhaps this can be expanded. What about retail activities, office space, or classrooms? I don't have the answer right now. But, working together, it behooves the region's leaders to find an appropriate use for this building. We owe it to our past, as well as to our future.

Note: The Landmark Society of Greater Utica formed an Old Main Re-Development Advisory Committee and is looking into ways to save the beautiful building, which is fondly viewed and cherished by many. Hopefully, the grand Doric columns will still be standing one hundred years from now. Patient care for the mentally ill continues on the Utica campus as Mohawk Valley Psychiatric Center offers inpatient and outpatient services for children and adults. Old Main is designated a national landmark and will continue to draw crowds to its grandeur and beauty.

Bibliography

American Journal of Insanity 1 (1844).

American Journal of Insanity 3 (1846).

American Phrenological Journal 9 (1847).

Annual Report of the Managers of the State Lunatic Asylum. Albany, NY: Argus Company Printers, 1869.

Batavia New York Spirit of the Times. "Horatio Ballard Secretary of State." May 23, 1863.

Brigham, Amariah, MD. "The Moral Treatment of the Insane." *American Journal of Insanity* 3 (1846).

Browne, W.A.F., Surgeon, *What Asylums Were, Are, and Ought to Be: Being the Substance of Five Lectures Delivered Before the Managers of the Montrose Royal Lunatic Asylum*. Edinburgh: Adam & Charles Black, 1852.

Clark, Lucy, and George M. White. *A Century of Progress at Utica State Hospital 1843–1943*. Utica, NY: 1943.

Dwyer, Ellen. *Homes for the Mad: Life Inside Two Nineteenth-Century Asylums*. New Brunswick, NJ: Rutgers University Press, 1987.

Familiar Views of Lunacy and Lunatic Life. London: John W. Parker Publisher, 1850.

Foucault, Michel. *Madness and Civilization: A History of Insanity in the Age of Reason*. New York: Pantheon Books, 1964.

Gaillard, E.S., MD. *Gaillard's Medical Journal*, Vol. 31. New York: A.G. Sherwood Printers, 1881.

Hale, Sarah Josepha. *Mrs. Hale's Receipts for the Million Containing Four Thousand Five Hundred and Forty-Five Receipts, Facts, Directions, Etc. in the Useful, Ornamental, And Domestic Arts, and in the Conduct of Life*. Philadelphia: T.B. Peterson, 1857.

Havana New York Journal. "News Alert." December 4, 1886.

Hitchcock, Henry Russell. *Architecture: Nineteenth and Twentieth Centuries*. New Haven, CT: Yale University Press, 1977.

Howard, Brian J. "What Is to Happen to Old Main?" Oneida County Historical Society, Utica, NY, 2015.

Jones, Pomroy. *Annals and Recollections of Oneida County*. Rome, NY: Published by author, 1851.

The Journal (Lowville, NY). "Burning of the State Lunatic Asylum." July 22, 1857.

Keene, Michael T. *Mad House: The Hidden History of Insane Asylums in 19th Century New York*. Fredericksburg, VA: Willow Manor Publishing, 2013.

Leech, John, MD. *Suggestions on the Law of Lunacy and Lunatic Asylums*, 2nd edition. Glasgow: John Churchill Publishers, 1852.

Mohawk Valley Psychiatric Center staff. *Mohawk Valley Psychiatric Center, 150 Years of Care*. Utica, NY: 1993.

New York Daily Tribune. "The Case of Speirs." July 28, 1857.

———. "The Case of William Speirs and the Fire." March 2, 1882.

———. "The State Lunatic Asylum Editorial." July 25, 1857.

New York Herald. "A Crying Disgrace—Ill Treatment of the Insane in New York State—The Utica Crib—A Barbarous Device for Restraining Unruly Patients—Strictness of Medical Experts—The Inspection of Asylums, as at Present Conduct, a Farce." November 23, 1879.

New York History Net. "Gerrit Smith—Harper's Ferry and the Aftermath." www.nyhistory.com/gerritsmith/harpers.htm.

Oneida (NY) *Weekly Herald and Gazette and Courier*. "The Asylum Fire." July 28, 1857.

Opal. A Monthly Periodical of the State Lunatic Asylum, Volumes 1–9, edited by the Patients, Utica, NY 1851–1859, 1959–1969. Oneida County History Center.

Penney, Darby, and Peter Stastny. *The Lives They Left Behind: Suitcases from a State Hospital Attic*. New York: Bellevue Literary Press, 2009.

Reiss, Benjamin. *Theaters of Madness: Insane Asylums & Nineteenth-Century American Culture*. Chicago: University of Chicago Press, 2008.

Rules, Regulations and By-Laws of the New York State Lunatic Asylum. Utica, NY: Ellis H. Roberts & Company, 1842, 1853.

Science Museum. Brought to Life: Exploring the History of Medicine. Philippe Pinel (1745-1826), www.sciencemuseum.org.uk/broughttolife/people/philippepinel.aspx.

Stuhler, Linda S. "The Care of the Insane in New York State (circa 1912)." VCU Libraries Social Welfare History Project. www.socialwelfarehistory.com/organizations/care-insane-new-york-1736-1912.

Trull, William L. *An Inner View of the State Lunatic Asylum at Utica or How Patients Are Treated in the Model Mad House of New York by William Trull an Ex-Patient*. Cohoes, NY: A. Craig, Printer, 1881.

Twelfth Report of the New York Civil Service Commission. Albany, NY: James B. Lyon Printer, 1895.

Weaver, Reverend G.S. *Lectures on Mental Science*. London: Fowlers and Wells Publishers, 1852.

Webster, Dennis, and Bernadette Peck. *Haunted Utica*. Charleston, SC: The History Press, 2014.

Acknowledgements

I want to thank the following, who gave me guidance, feedback and friendship in the creation of this book: George Abel; Michael Bosak; Andrew Buffington; Jeff Burman; Ellen Dwyer, PhD; Jim Folts; Rebecca McLain; Lou Parrotta; Carl Saporito; Banks Smither, The History Press; Landmark Society; Old Fulton Postcards; Oneida County Historical Center; New York State Archives; and Utica Public Library.

About the Author

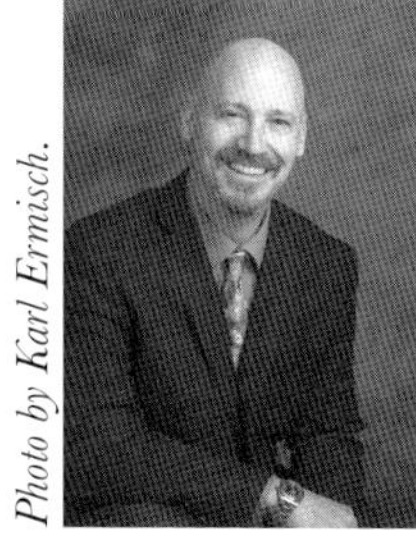
Photo by Karl Ermisch.

Dennis Webster lives in the midst of the Mohawk Valley of Central New York, not far from the steadfast pillars of Old Main. He has a Bachelor of Science degree from Utica College and a Master of Business Administration (MBA) degree from the State University of New York (SUNY) Polytechnic. He's the author of paranormal—*Haunted Utica*, *Haunted Mohawk Valley*, *Haunted Old Forge*—and true crime books, *Wicked Adirondacks*, *Wicked Mohawk Valley* and *Murder of a Herkimer County Teacher*. He can be reached at denniswbstr@gmail.com.